WORKBOOK AND LICENSURE EXAM PREP FOR RADIOGRAPHY ESSENTIALS
FOR LIMITED PRACTICE

WORKBOOK AND LICENSURE EXAM PREP FOR RADIOGRAPHY ESSENTIALS

FOR LIMITED PRACTICE

Fifth Edition

BRUCE W. LONG
MS, RT(R)(CV), FASRT, FAEIRS
Director and Associate Professor
Radiologic and Imaging Sciences Programs
Indiana University School of Medicine
Indianapolis, Indiana

EUGENE D. FRANK
MA, RT(R), FASRT, FAEIRS
Associate Professor Emeritus
Mayo Clinic College of Medicine
Rochester, Minnesota

RUTH ANN EHRLICH
RT(R)
Retired, Radiology Faculty
University of Western States
Portland, Oregon;
Adjunct Faculty
Portland Community College
Portland, Oregon

Contributing Author

SHARON R. WARTENBEE
RT(R)(BD), CBDT, FASRT
Senior Diagnostic and Bone Densitometry
Technologist
Avera Medical Group McGreevy
Sioux Falls, South Dakota

ELSEVIER

ELSEVIER

3251 Riverport Lane
St. Louis, Missouri 63043

Workbook and Licensure Exam Prep for Radiography Essentials
for Limited Practice, FIFTH EDITION

ISBN: 978-0-323459587

Notices

Knowledge and best practice in this field are constantly changing. As new research and experience broaden our understanding, changes in research methods, professional practices, or medical treatment may become necessary.

Practitioners and researchers must always rely on their own experience and knowledge in evaluating and using any information, methods, compounds, or experiments described herein. In using such information or methods they should be mindful of their own safety and the safety of others, including parties for whom they have a professional responsibility.

With respect to any drug or pharmaceutical products identified, readers are advised to check the most current information provided (i) on procedures featured or (ii) by the manufacturer of each product to be administered, to verify the recommended dose or formula, the method and duration of administration, and contraindications. It is the responsibility of practitioners, relying on their own experience and knowledge of their patients, to make diagnoses, to determine dosages and the best treatment for each individual patient, and to take all appropriate safety precautions.

To the fullest extent of the law, neither the Publisher nor the authors, contributors, or editors, assume any liability for any injury and/or damage to persons or property as a matter of products liability, negligence or otherwise, or from any use or operation of any methods, products, instructions, or ideas contained in the material herein.

Content Strategist: Sonya Seigafuse
Content Development Manager: Billie C. Sharp
Content Development Specialist: Laurel Shea
Publishing Services Manager: Hemamalini Rajendrababu
Project Manager: Radhika Sivalingam
Cover Designer: Muthukumaran Thangaraj

Printed in the United States of America

Last digit is the print number: 9 8 7 6 5 4 3 2 1

Working together
to grow libraries in
developing countries

www.elsevier.com • www.bookaid.org

Contents

Answers to Section I can be found on the Evolve site at http://evolve.elsevier.com/Long/radiographylimited.

1 Role of the Limited X-ray Machine Operator

EXERCISE 1

Answer the following questions by selecting the best choice.

1. X-rays were discovered by:
   A. Eastman.
   B. Crookes.
   C. Edison.
   D. Roentgen.

2. The Joint Review Committee on Education in Radiologic Technology (JRCERT) is the:
   A. organization that accredits schools for radiologic technologists.
   B. organization that accredits schools for limited operators.
   C. professional organization for radiologic technologists.
   D. professional organization for limited operators.

3. Another term that has the same meaning as *practical radiographer* is:
   A. radiologic technologist.
   B. medical assistant.
   C. limited operator.
   D. imaging specialist.

4. (True/False) To determine the credentials needed for you to practice limited radiography, you should contact the appropriate state agency.

5. The term *limited* operator is used because the:
   A. scope of practice is limited.
   B. salaries are limited.
   C. opportunities are limited.
   D. radiographer's competence is limited.

6. *Reciprocity* means that:
   A. special credentials are required.
   B. credentials issued in one area are recognized in another.
   C. an application has been made for a license or permit but the license or permit has not been granted.
   D. there is freedom to practice without a license or permit.

7. Which of the following physicians has received extensive additional training and would be considered a specialist?
   1. Radiologist
   2. Obstetrician
   3. Pediatrician
   A. 1 and 2
   B. 1 and 3
   C. 2 and 3
   D. 1, 2, and 3

8. A specialist who interprets radiographs and performs special imaging procedures is called:
   A. a radiologic technologist.
   B. a chiropractor.
   C. a primary care physician.
   D. a radiologist.

9. An order for an x-ray examination is issued by:
   A. a physician.
   B. a nurse.
   C. a radiologic technologist.
   D. a medical assistant.

10. Which of the following are considered duties of a limited operator?
    1. Determine what examination should be performed.
    2. Explain the procedure and the preparation to the patient.
    3. Position the patient correctly in relation to the image receptor and the x-ray tube.
    A. 1 and 2
    B. 1 and 3
    C. 2 and 3
    D. 1, 2, and 3

11. The largest professional organization for radiologic technologists is the:
    A. ARRT.
    B. ASRT.
    C. JRCERT.
    D. ASSRT.

12. The curriculum for limited x-ray machine operators is published by the:
    A. ARRT.
    B. ASRT.
    C. JRCERT.
    D. ASSRT.

13. An organization that now provides accreditation for limited x-ray schools is the:
    A. ARRT.
    B. ASRT.
    C. JRCERT.
    D. ASSRT.

14. A podiatrist diagnoses and treats disorders and diseases of:
    A. the chest.
    B. the feet.
    C. children.
    D. the nervous system.

15. Bone densitometry is a specialized x-ray machine and procedure that measures:
    A. bone growth.
    B. bone mineral content.
    C. bone aging.
    D. bone blood flow.

16. Which of the following documents cites information that is "mandatory and enforceable"?
    A. ARRT Code of Ethics
    B. ARRT Rules of Ethics
    C. ARRT Handbook
    D. ARRT Standard of Ethics

17. (True/False) Limited operators can perform the same x-ray examinations that radiographers can.

18. (True/False) Credentials for limited operators vary greatly from state to state.

EXERCISE 2

Answer the following questions.

1. When, where, and by whom were x-rays discovered?

_____

_____

2. What is the purpose of the ARRT? Why might this organization be important to a limited x-ray machine operator?

_____

_____

_____

3. List the possible consequences of practicing radiography outside the limitations imposed by local regulations.

_____

_____

_____

_____

4. What is the professional credential used by radiologic technologists after passing the ARRT examination in radiography, and what does it stand for?

_____

_____

5. Explain what is meant by *reciprocity*.

_____

_____

6. List three activities that might take place in the "front office" of a clinic and four that typically occur in the "back office."

   Front office:

   1. _____

   2. _____

   3. _____

   Back office:

   1. _____

   2. _____

   3. _____

   4. _____

7. List five typical duties of a limited x-ray machine operator.

   1. _____

   2. _____

   3. _____

   4. _____

   5. _____

8. The official term for people who perform limited x-ray procedures is *limited x-ray machine operator.* Name at least three other terms that may be used in some states.

   1. _____

   2. _____

   3. _____

Answer the following questions.

1. How can you determine the location of the central ray?

   _____

   _____

2. What is the location of remnant radiation?

   _____

   _____

3. What is meant by *attenuation?*

   _____

   _____

4. What component of the x-ray machine is located in the control booth?

   _____

   _____

5. What should you do before attempting to move x-ray equipment?

   _____

   _____

6. Where would you look to find a collimator?

   _____

   _____

7. How might you determine the size of the radiation field without actually measuring it?

   _____

   _____

8. List the four steps in a pre-exposure safety check.

   1. _____

   2. _____

   3. _____

   4. _____

9. How soon is it safe to re-enter the x-ray room after an exposure?

_____

_____

10. Define the difference between primary and remnant radiation.

_____

_____

_____

_____

11. What are the common sizes of CR plates?

_____

12. Describe the Trendelenburg position.

_____

_____

13. Describe the latent image.

_____

_____

14. Many x-ray projections are done with the patient standing or sitting upright using what device?

_____

EXERCISE 3

Match the following terms with their descriptions.

1. _____ Tube housing

2. _____ Tube port

3. _____ X-ray tube

4. _____ Scatter radiation

5. _____ Radiation fog

6. _____ Computed radiography (CR)

7. _____ Image receptor (IR)

A. Source of the x-rays

B. Unwanted image exposure that is caused by scattered x-rays

C. Surrounds the x-ray tube and is lined with lead

D. Filmless x-ray system that uses a digital format to produce images

E. Receives the energy of the x-ray beam and forms the image of the body part

F. Opening where the x-rays exit the tube

G. The x-rays that strike the patient and travel in all directions, inside and outside the body

CHALLENGE EXERCISE

This exercise does not have to be completed at the same time as the other exercises in this workbook chapter. The exercise is designed to assess retention of the essential information contained in the corresponding textbook chapter. It is recommended that you complete this exercise when you begin to study for the state limited licensure examination. This will help determine what you know and which information should be further reviewed.

1. X-rays exit the tube port through an opening called the:

   _____.

2. The x-ray tube is surrounded by a lead-lined device called the:

   _____.

3. The invisible imaginary line in the center of the x-ray beam that is used for centering is called the:

   _____.

4. The square lighted area on the patient and table where the x-rays strike is called the:

   _____.

5. What is the name of the radiation that exits the patient?

   _____.

6. The unseen image contained within the plate phosphor is called the:

   _____.

7. The x-ray beam that leaves the tube is called:

   _____.

8. The absorption of x-rays by the human body is called:

   _____.

9. The primary source of scatter radiation is the:

   _____.

10. Primary-beam x-rays that leave the body and travel in all directions are called:

    _____.

11. What is the difference in energy between the primary-beam radiation and the scattered radiation?

    _____.

12. The unwanted radiation exposure on the x-ray image caused by scatter radiation is called:

    _____.

13. Scatter radiation exits the patient in which direction?

_____

14. In the radiology department today, the IR consists of what two components?

_____

15. Which digital imaging system do most limited operators use today?

_____

16. What is the name of the device that accepts the CR plate and scans it?

_____

17. The most frequent adverse incident that occurs in the radiology department is:

_____

18. Name several key safety precautions that should occur when moving x-ray equipment.

_____

19. What is the name of the movable device under the x-ray table that contains a grid and holds the IR?

_____

20. The device that allows x-rays to be taken in the upright position is called the:

_____

21. Lowering the head on the x-ray table at least 15 degrees is termed:

_____

22. Name several important pre-exposure safety checks:

_____

3 Basic Mathematics for Limited Operators

EXERCISE 1

Match the following terms with their definitions.

1. _____ Sum

2. _____ Difference

3. _____ Product

4. _____ Dividend

5. _____ Divisor

6. _____ Quotient

7. _____ Remainder

A. The number that is "left over" when the dividend cannot be evenly divided by the divisor

B. The answer to a multiplication problem

C. Total, the answer to an addition problem

D. The number by which the dividend is divided

E. The answer to a division problem

F. The answer to a subtraction problem

G. In a division problem, the number that is divided

EXERCISE 2

Answer the following questions.

1. The lower number of a fraction is called the _____.

2. The upper number of a fraction is called the _____.

3. A mixed number consists of a(n)_____ and a(n)_____.

4. To multiply a whole number by a fraction, multiply the whole number by

_____ and then divide the product by

_____.

5. Calculate the value of the following fractions of whole numbers.

    A. $\frac{1}{10} \times 80$ _____

    B. $\frac{1}{10} \times 200$ _____

    C. $\frac{2}{5} \times 150$ _____

    D. $\frac{1}{4} \times 300$ _____

    E. $\frac{7}{10} \times 80$ _____

6. Reduce the following fractions to the lowest terms.

A. $\frac{4}{10}$ _____

B. $\frac{3}{12}$ _____

C. $\frac{6}{18}$ _____

D. $\frac{12}{20}$ _____

E. $\frac{8}{24}$ _____

F. $\frac{15}{25}$ _____

G. $\frac{6}{8}$ _____

EXERCISE 3

Answer the following questions.

1. In a decimal, numerals to the left of the decimal point represent _____.

2. The first place to the right of the decimal point represents _____, the second place represents _____

_____, and the third place represents _____.

3. (True/False) 0.7 = 0.700.

4. (True/False) 3.3 = 3.03.

5. Set up the problems and calculate the sums of the following decimals.

A. 21.7 + 5.39 = _____.

B. 33.06 + 30.2 = _____.

C. 14.911 + 208.7 = _____.

D. 29.844 + 3.3 + 27.6 = _____.

E. $285.2 + 46.91 + 11.402 =$ _____.

6. Set up the problems and calculate the differences of the following decimals.

   A. $335.65 - 46.23 =$ _____.

   B. $456.33 - 3.87 =$ _____.

   C. $39.8 - 6.323 =$ _____.

   D. $21 - 7.51 =$ _____.

   E. $19.042 - 4.12 =$ _____.

7. How do you determine where to place the decimal point in a problem that involves multiplication of decimals?

   _____

   _____

8. Set up the problems and calculate the products in the following problems involving multiplication of decimals.

A. $29.5 \times 5 =$ _____.

B. $17.6 \times 40 =$ _____.

C. $341.225 \times 48.33 =$ _____.

D. $0.2213 \times 82.7 =$ _____.

E. $83.22 \times 906.1 =$ _____.

9. Set up the problems and calculate the quotients in the following problems involving division of decimals.

A. $34.5 \div 5 =$ _____.

B. $720.35 \div 10 =$ _____.

C. $29 \div 2.5 =$ _____.

D. $284.31 \div 4.05 =$ _____.

E. $609.56 \div 6.22 =$ _____.

Chapter **3**   **Basic Mathematics for Limited Operators**

10. To convert a fraction to a decimal, divide the ______________________ by the ______________________.

11. Convert the following fractions and mixed numbers to decimals.

A. $\frac{1}{8}$ ______________________

B. $\frac{3}{8}$ ______________________

C. $\frac{1}{60}$ ______________________

D. $\frac{2}{5}$ ______________________

E. $1\frac{1}{4}$ ______________________

12. *(Circle the correct phrase.)* When rounding off a decimal, drop the excess numerals from (left to right/right to left).

13. When rounding off a decimal, if the last numeral dropped is ______________ or greater, increase the final remaining numeral by one; if the last numeral dropped is ______________ or less, no change is necessary.

14. Round off the following decimals to the number of decimal places indicated in parentheses.

A. 1.66666 (2) ______________________

B. 0.74139 (4) ______________________

C. 0.2509 (2) ______________________

D. 3.2551 (3) ______________________

E. 10.4444 (2) ______________________

15. Perform the indicated calculations in the following problems by first converting the fractions to decimals. If the decimals in this exercise have four or more decimal places, round them off to three decimal places.

A. $\frac{1}{4} + \frac{1}{20} + \frac{2}{3} =$ ______________________.

B. $\frac{3}{10} + \frac{1}{5} + \frac{1}{2} =$ ______________________.

C. $\frac{3}{4} - \frac{3}{8} =$ ______________________.

D. $\frac{2}{15} \times 200 =$ ______________________.

E. $\frac{3}{5} \div \frac{1}{2} =$ ______________________.

EXERCISE 4

Answer the following questions.

1. (True/False) When adding or subtracting two percentages, the percentages must be converted to decimals.

2. (True/False) When multiplying or dividing percentages, or when performing calculations involving percentages and whole numbers, the percentages must be converted to decimals.

3. Convert the following percentages to decimals.

    A. 20% _____

    B. 71.3% _____

    C. 85% _____

    D. 69% _____

    E. 172% _____

    F. 800% _____

4. Convert the following decimals to percentages.

    A. 0.33 _____

    B. 0.4 _____

    C. 0.06 _____

    D. 1.89 _____

    E. 2.3 _____

    F. 6.0 _____

5. Perform the following calculations involving percentages.

    A. 73% + 27% = _____.

    B. 50% + 25% = _____.

    C. 30% − 3% = _____.

    D. 20% × 60% = _____.

    E. 79% × 30% = _____.

    F. 25% ÷ 10% = _____.

    G. 48% ÷ 2% = _____.

6. Calculate the values of the following percentages up to two decimal places.

    A. 30% of 27 = _____.

    B. 95% of 320 = _____.

C. 50% of 31 = _____.

D. 170% of 60 = _____.

E. 200% of 20 = _____.

7. Determine the following percentages. Express your answers to the nearest tenth of a percent.

A. 11 = _____% of 64

B. 71 = _____% of 90

C. 50 = _____% of 300

D. 40 = _____% of 200

E. 70 = _____% of 35

Chapter **3** **Basic Mathematics for Limited Operators**

8. Calculate the solutions to the following problems that involve increasing and decreasing numbers by a percentage.

   A. Increase 75 by 15%.

   B. Increase 30 by 100%.

   C. Increase 12 by 20%.

   D. Decrease 85 by 10%.

   E. Decrease 50 by 12%.

Answer the following questions.

1. A declaration that two mathematical statements (groups of numbers, together with their operational signs or mathematical functions) are equal to each other is called a(n) _____.

2. (True/False) The same symbols for mathematical operations used in arithmetic are also used in algebra.

3. *(Circle the correct word.)* The slanted line between the x and the 3 in the equation $x/3 = 6$ means that x is (multiplied/divided) by 3.

4. (True/False) When an equation consists of two fractions, you can eliminate the denominators from consideration by using cross multiplication.

5. 3:4 is an example of a(n)_____.

6. 3:4::6:8 is an example of a(n)_____.

7. Determine the value of x up to three decimal places in each of the following equations.

   A. $2x + 9 = 11 + 3$

   B. $16/x = 12 - 4$

   C. $x - 61 = 12$

   D. $45 = 4x - 15$

   E. $3x = 2/3$

   F. $64 = 8x$

G. $\frac{25}{x} = \frac{10}{2}$

H. $\frac{x}{3} = \frac{48}{12}$

I. $\frac{72}{8} = \frac{80}{x}$

J. $\frac{10}{x} = \frac{4}{6}$

EXERCISE 6

Answer the following questions.

1. Write the expression that indicates four cubed. _____

2. Write the expression that indicates five to the fifth power. _____

3. Calculate the values of the following exponential numbers.

A. $3^2 = $ _____.

B. $3^3 = $ _____.

C. $2^4 = $ _____.

D. $9^2 = $ _____.

E. $40^2 =$ _____.

4. Calculate the square roots in the following problems.

A. $\sqrt{9} =$ _____.

B. $\sqrt{16} =$ _____.

C. $\sqrt{25} =$ _____.

D. $\sqrt{81} =$ _____.

E. $\sqrt{144} =$ _____.

EXERCISE 7

1. Match the metric prefixes with their meanings.

1. _____ Kilo-	A. 10
2. _____ Nano-	B. 100
3. _____ Milli-	C. 1000
4. _____ Deci-	D. $\frac{1}{10}$ (0.1)
5. _____ Hecto-	E. $\frac{1}{100}$ (0.01)
6. _____ Centi-	F. $\frac{1}{1000}$ (0.001)
7. _____ Micro-	G. $\frac{1}{1,000,000}$ (0.000001)
8. _____ Deka-	H. $\frac{1}{1,000,000,000}$ (0.000000001)

2. Fill in the blanks in these statements of English measurement equivalents.

A. One yard = _____ feet.

B. One foot = _____ inches.

C. One pint = _____ ounces.

D. One ton = _____ pounds.

E. One pound = _____ ounces.

3. Fill in the blanks in these statements of metric equivalents.

    A. 1 meter = _____ centimeters.

    B. 1 kilogram = _____ grams.

    C. 1 liter = _____ milliliters.

    D. 1 millisecond = _____ second.

4. Convert the following metric measurements from one unit to another.

    A. Convert 70 kilovolts to volts.

    B. Convert 5 meters to centimeters.

    C. Convert 30 milliliters to liters.

    D. Convert 100 grams to kilograms.

    E. Convert 2 milligrams to grams.

5. Convert the following measurements from one English unit to another.

    A. Convert 18 inches to yards.

    B. Convert 2 quarts to fluid ounces.

    C. Convert 68 inches to feet.

D. Convert 20 quarts to gallons.

E. Convert 3.5 pounds to ounces.

6. Calculate the following conversions between English and metric units. Limit your answers to no more than four decimal places.

A. Convert 5 fluid ounces to milliliters.

B. Convert 100 pounds to kilograms.

C. Convert 14 inches to meters.

D. Convert 50 millimeters to inches.

E. Convert 100 grams to ounces.

7. Calculate the following time and temperature conversions.

A. Convert $\frac{1}{60}$ second to milliseconds.

B. Convert 260 seconds to hours.

C. Convert 2.4 days to hours.

D. Convert 75° F to the Celsius scale.

E. Convert 25° C to the Fahrenheit scale.

EXERCISE 8

Answer the following questions.

1. Milliampere-seconds (mAs) is a useful unit in radiography because it indicates _____.

2. State the formula for determining mAs. _____.

3. When both mA and mAs are known, the formula for determining the exposure time is _____

_____.

4. Calculate the mAs for the following exposures.

    A. 200 mA, 0.05 second

    B. 300 mA, 0.25 second

    C. 100 mA, 0.7 second

    D. 500 mA, ½₀ second

    E. 50 mA, 0.3 second

F. 150 mA, 1¼ seconds

G. 400 mA, 2 milliseconds

5. Calculate the exposure time for the following exposures. Round any extended decimals to three decimal places.

A. 50 mA, 10 mAs

B. 200 mA, 40 mAs

C. 300 mA, 6 mAs

D. 100 mA, 2 mAs

E. 400 mA, 75 mAs

EXERCISE 9

Answer the following questions.

1. Write the formula for changing mAs to compensate for a change in source–image receptor distance (SID).

   _____

2. Solve the following problems involving changes in SID.

   A. What is the relative change in radiation intensity when the distance changes from 40 inches SID to 80 inches SID?

B. What is the relative change in radiation intensity when the distance is changed from 60 inches SID to 40 inches SID?

C. A satisfactory radiograph is made using 25 mAs at 40 inches SID. How many mAs are needed to produce a similar radiograph at 48 inches SID?

D. A satisfactory radiograph is made using 30 mAs at 72 inches SID. How many mAs are needed to produce a similar radiograph at 84 inches SID?

E. A satisfactory radiograph is made using 12 mAs at 40 inches SID. How many mAs are needed to produce a similar radiograph at 72 inches SID?

EXERCISE 10

Answer the following questions.

1. Below 85 peak kilovoltage (kVp), an adjustment of _____ kVp/cm will compensate for small changes in part

   size. Above 85 kVp, a change of _____ kVp/cm is necessary.

2. To compensate for a 2-cm *increase* in part size using mAs, increase the original mAs by _____%. To compen-

   sate for a 2-cm *decrease* in part size using mAs, decrease the original mAs by _____%.

3. Solve the following problems involving changes in patient part size.

   A. A satisfactory radiograph is made using 90 kVp on a patient part measuring 24 cm. Adjust the kVp to compensate for a patient part size decrease to 21 cm.

   B. A satisfactory radiograph is made using 72 kVp on a patient part measuring 16 cm. Adjust the kVp to compensate for a patient part size increase to 19 cm.

C. A satisfactory radiograph is made using 20 mAs on a patient part measuring 22 cm. Adjust the mAs to compensate for a patient part size decrease to 20 cm.

D. A satisfactory radiograph is made using 50 mAs on a patient part measuring 26 cm. Adjust the mAs to compensate for a patient part size increase to 30 cm.

E. A satisfactory radiograph is made using 15 mAs on a patient part measuring 13 cm. Adjust the mAs to compensate for a patient part size increase to 15 cm.

EXERCISE 11

Answer the following questions.

1. *(Circle the correct word.)* The kVp is (increased/decreased) to shorten the scale of contrast.

2. *(Circle the correct word.)* When using the 15% rule to increase kVp, you must (multiply/divide) the mAs by 2.

3. Solve the following problems using the 15% rule.

   A. An exposure made using 20 mAs and 95 kVp has a satisfactory radiographic density. Suggest a new technique that will provide more contrast.

   B. An exposure made using 120 mAs and 78 kVp has a satisfactory radiographic density. Suggest a new technique that will decrease the patient dose.

C. An exposure made using 20 mAs and 60 kVp has a satisfactory radiographic density. Suggest a new technique that will provide more latitude.

D. An exposure made using 25 mAs and 100 kVp has a satisfactory radiographic density. Suggest a new technique that will provide more contrast.

E. An exposure made using 30 mAs and 70 kVp has a satisfactory radiographic density. Suggest a new technique that will provide less contrast.

EXERCISE 12

Answer the following questions.

1. Write the formula used for determining the volume of medication that will deliver a specific dose. _____

   _____

2. The prescribed dose is 60 mg. The available stock is in the form of 15-mg tablets. How many should be given?

3. The prescribed dose is 150 mg. The available stock has a strength of 50 mg/mL. How much should be given?

4. The prescribed dose is 80 mcg. The available stock has a strength of 20 mcg/mL. How much should be given?

5. The prescribed dose is 2 mg. The available stock has a strength of 1 mg per tablet. How much should be given?

6. A toddler got into the medicine cabinet and ate four acetaminophen (Tylenol) tablets. The tablet strength is 500 mg. What dose did the child receive?

7. A physician prescribed a dose of 2 mg/kg of body weight for a child. The child weighs 40 pounds. The drug is available in a strength of 4 mg/mL. How many milliliters should the child receive?

CHALLENGE EXERCISE

This exercise does not have to be completed at the same time as the other exercises in this workbook chapter. The exercise is designed to assess retention of the essential information contained in the corresponding textbook chapter. It is recommended that you complete this exercise when you begin to study for the state limited licensure examination. This will help determine what you know and which information should be further reviewed.

1. The answer to a division problem is called the _____.

2. Calculate the result when 85 is increased by 15%. _____

3. If the mAs are increased from 20 to 30, what is the percentage of the increase? _____

4. The factor that indicates the total quantity of radiation in an exposure is the _____.

5. An exposure is made using 500 mAs and 3 msec. Calculate the mAs for this exposure.

   _____

6. How many milliliters are contained in a liter? _____

7. An exposure made using 10 mAs and 90 kVp has a satisfactory radiographic density. Suggest a new technique that will provide more contrast.

   _____

8. The prescribed dose of a drug is 120 mcg. The available stock has a strength of 20 mcg/mL. What quantity should be given?

   _____

9. State the formula for determining the new mAs to compensate for a change in SID.

   _____

4 Basic Physics for Radiography

Answer the following questions by selecting the best choice.

1. Which of the following would be considered a basic form of matter?
   1. Solid
   2. Liquid
   3. Mass
   A. 1 and 2
   B. 1 and 3
   C. 2 and 3
   D. 1, 2, and 3

2. The quantity of matter that makes up any physical object is called the:
   A. nucleus.
   B. atomic number.
   C. mass.
   D. energy.

3. Which of the following is located in an orbit around the nucleus of an atom?
   A. Photon
   B. Electron
   C. Neutron
   D. Positron

4. Which of the following has a negative (−) electrical charge?
   A. Neutron
   B. Proton
   C. Electron
   D. Positron

5. Which of the following are considered fundamental particles of atoms?
   1. Neutrons
   2. Photons
   3. Protons
   A. 1 and 2
   B. 1 and 3
   C. 2 and 3
   D. 1, 2, and 3

6. When a neutral atom gains or loses an electron, the atom is said to be:
   A. radioactive.
   B. unstable.
   C. ionized.
   D. neutral.

7. Mechanical energy can be classified as either kinetic energy or:
   A. magnetic energy.
   B. electromagnetic energy.
   C. chemical energy.
   D. potential energy.

8. X-rays consist of:
   A. electromagnetic energy.
   B. potential energy.
   C. chemical energy.
   D. thermal energy.

9. X-rays with greater energy have a shorter _____ and are more penetrating.
   A. frequency
   B. velocity
   C. wavelength
   D. potential difference

10. Of the following types of electromagnetic energy, which has the shortest wavelength?
    A. Radio waves
    B. Diagnostic rays
    C. Microwaves
    D. Ultraviolet light

11. Which of the following are accurate statements regarding the characteristics of x-rays?
    1. They are highly penetrating and invisible.
    2. They cause certain crystals to fluoresce.
    3. They travel in straight lines at the speed of light.
    A. 1 and 2
    B. 1 and 3
    C. 2 and 3
    D. 1, 2, and 3

12. The smallest possible unit of electromagnetic energy is the:
    A. photon.
    B. atom.
    C. nuclear energy.
    D. matter.

13. The term for a continuous path for the flow of electrical charges from the power source through one or more electrical devices and back to the source is:
    A. electrical circuit.
    B. voltage.
    C. frequency.
    D. resistance.

8. An exposure is made using 100 mA and 0.25 seconds. What is the value of the mAs? State another combination of mA and time that will produce the same quantity of exposure.

_____

_____

_____

9. If the x-ray tube has 0.5 mm Al equiv inherent filtration, and the collimator provides an additional 1.25 mm Al equiv, how much filtration must be added to meet minimum safety requirements?

_____

10. What is the standard rotation speed of the x-ray tube's anode?

_____

11. What is the percentage of characteristic radiation that is produced below 70 kVp?

_____

12. What is the difference in radiation intensity between the anode and cathode ends of the x-ray beam when a 14- × 17-inch IR is used at a 40-inch SID (state in percentage)?

_____

13. The primary purpose of filtration is to:

_____

14. Name the three components of the x-ray tube that contribute to the inherent filtration.

1. _____

2. _____

3. _____

EXERCISE 3

Label the following drawings.

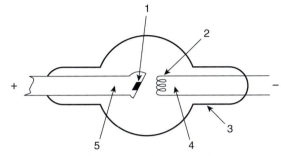

FIG. 5.1 Simple x-ray tube.

1. _____

2. _____

3. _____

4. _____

5. _____

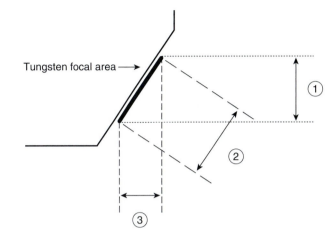

 Film

FIG. 5.2 Effective focal spot.

1. _____

2. _____

3. _____

EXERCISE 4

Find the mAs for each of the technical factors below.

1. 20 mA × 1.00 sec = _____ mAs

2. 10 mA × 0.50 sec = _____ mAs

3. 100 mA × 0.75 sec = _____ mAs

4. 50 mA × 1.50 sec = _____ mAs

Determine the mA for each of the mAs values below.

5. 100 mAs = _____ mA × 2.00 sec

6. 200 mAs = _____ mA × 0.50 sec

7. 300 mAs = _____ mA × 1.50 sec

8. 75 mAs = _____ mA × 0.75 sec

Find the seconds for each of the mAs and mA values below.

9. 100 mAs = 100 mA × _____ sec

10. 200 mAs = 400 mA × _____ sec

11. 500 mAs = 250 mA × _____ sec

12. 300 mAs = 400 mA × _____ sec

CHALLENGE EXERCISE

This exercise does not have to be completed at the same time as the other exercises in this workbook chapter. The exercise is designed to assess retention of the essential information contained in the corresponding textbook chapter. It is recommended that you complete this exercise when you begin to study for the state limited licensure examination. This will help determine what you know and which information should be further reviewed.

1. Of what material is the filament made?

   _____

2. Of what material is the target/anode made?

   _____

3. What is added to the port to remove the long-wavelength radiation?

   _____

4. What is the term used to describe the heating of an element to a hot temperature and the expanding of the electrons in the atom?

   _____

5. Is the cathode side of the x-ray tube positive or negative?

   _____

6. Is the anode side of the x-ray tube positive or negative?

   _____

7. What is the purpose of having a "high-speed" anode?

   _____

8. What are the two rotation speeds for the anode?

   _____

9. What type of radiation production makes up the greatest portion of the x-ray beam—bremsstrahlung or characteristic?

   _____

10. Characteristic radiation is not produced below which kVp level?

_____

11. The majority of the energy in the x-ray tube is converted to:

_____

12. What is the name of the radiation produced when an incoming electron into the anode is suddenly braked and deviated?

_____

13. The degree of angulation of the x-ray tube target (anode) will determine the:

_____

14. How is the volume or intensity of x-rays affected by the heel effect?

_____

15. To take advantage of the heel effect on a body part that has both a thick area and a thin area, where should the cathode be placed?

_____

16. The power and speed of the electrons inside the x-ray tube and the energy of the x-rays that emerge are controlled by the:

_____

17. The current, or volume, of x-ray production is measured in units of:

_____

18. The mA or mAs used for an exposure determines the:

_____

19. The penetrating power of the x-ray beam is controlled by the:

_____

20. Name two characteristics of tungsten.

_____

21. How much aluminum filtration must be in the x-ray tube to meet government standards?

_____

22. What is the advantage of using aluminum filtration in the port of the x-ray tube?

_____

23. Name the three components that make up the inherent filtration.

_____

24. The amount of detail or resolution seen in the radiographic image is referred to as:

_____.

25. What type of motor is used to turn the anode inside the x-ray tube?

_____

26. When is the large focal spot used?

_____

27. The anode heel effect is most pronounced when using which size of IR?

_____

6 X-ray Circuit and Tube Heat Management

EXERCISE 1

Answer the following questions by selecting the best choice.

1. All of the following devices are located within the low-voltage circuit and control console *except* the:
   A. step-up transformer.
   B. kilovolt control.
   C. exposure switch.
   D. autotransformer.

2. The autotransformer's primary purpose is to vary the:
   A. voltage.
   B. amperage.
   C. exposure time.
   D. high frequency.

3. Which transformer is located in the filament circuit?
   A. Rectifier
   B. Step-up transformer
   C. Step-down transformer
   D. Autotransformer

4. The primary purpose of the filament circuit is to:
   A. control the exposure time.
   B. supply voltage to the x-ray tube.
   C. heat the x-ray tube filament for thermionic emission.
   D. supply power to the autotransformer.

5. A timer that is capable of producing ultrashort exposure times is typical of a(n):
   A. electronic timer.
   B. synchronous (impulse) timer.
   C. mechanical timer.
   D. phototimer.

6. The primary purpose of a rectifier in an x-ray circuit is to:
   A. vary the peak kilovoltage (kVp).
   B. vary the milliamperes (mA).
   C. measure current in the x-ray tube.
   D. change alternating current (AC) into direct current (DC).

7. The primary purpose of the high-voltage circuit is to:
   A. vary the kVp in the x-ray tube.
   B. supply the x-ray tube with voltage high enough to produce x-rays.
   C. change AC into DC.
   D. increase the frequency from 60 hertz (Hz) to 6000 Hz.

8. The advantages of using a high-frequency generator instead of a single-phase generator include:
   1. producing x-rays more efficiently.
   2. requiring less exposure time to produce a given amount of exposure.
   3. producing the greatest amount of x-rays for the same exposure technique.
   A. 1 and 2
   B. 1 and 3
   C. 2 and 3
   D. 1, 2, and 3

9. How much can the exposure time be decreased when using three-phase x-ray equipment?
   A. 20%
   B. 30%
   C. 40%
   D. 50% to 60%

10. Automatic exposure control (AEC) automatically varies the:
    A. mA.
    B. kVp.
    C. exposure time.
    D. mA and kVp.

11. If the automatic exposure control fails during the exposure, the _____ will terminate the exposure.
    A. rectifier
    B. high-voltage circuit
    C. filament circuit
    D. back-up timer

5. List two advantages of using a high-frequency x-ray generator compared with a single-phase or three-phase generator.

   1. _____

   2. _____

6. State, in order, the four steps for making an x-ray exposure after the control panel has been set.

   1. _____

   2. _____

   3. _____

   4. _____

7. Name two things that occur when the rotor switch is activated.

   1. _____

   2. _____

8. Name at least three features of an x-ray tube that are designed for handling the high heat.

   1. _____

   2. _____

   3. _____

9. To ensure that x-ray tubes will last a long time, the maximum heat capacity should remain below:

   _____.

10. If an exposure is made at 300 mA, 1 sec, and 90 kVp using a single-phase generator, how many heat units are generated at the anode?

   _____

11. Where is the center automatic exposure control detector located on a three-detector system?

   _____

12. The small focal spot is used when mA stations below _____ mA are used.

13. Name the three transformers in an x-ray machine.

   1. _____

   2. _____

   3. _____

14. Name at least five technical factors that are automatically set when using anatomically programmed radiography.

   1. _____

   2. _____

   3. _____

   4. _____

   5. _____

CHALLENGE EXERCISE

This exercise does not have to be completed at the same time as the other exercises in this workbook chapter. The exercise is designed to assess retention of the essential information contained in the corresponding textbook chapter. It is recommended that you complete this exercise when you begin to study for the state limited licensure examination. This will help determine what you know and which information should be further reviewed.

1. What are the names of the three x-ray circuits?

   _____

2. What is the purpose of the autotransformer?

   _____

3. What is the purpose of the filament circuit?

   _____

4. What is the purpose of the high-voltage circuit?

   _____

5. Name the three transformers used in the x-ray circuit.

   _____

6. In which circuit is the step-down transformer located?

   _____

7. In which circuit is the step-up transformer located?

   _____

8. The process of changing AC to DC is called:

   _____

9. How many pulses of radiation occur in a full-wave rectified x-ray machine?

   _____

10. What type of rectification is used in most modern x-ray generators?

_____

11. Name the three types of x-ray generators.

_____

12. Which x-ray generator has the lowest power?

_____

13. How much more x-ray output is achieved by using a three-phase x-ray generator?

_____

14. The most common x-ray generator used today is the:

_____.

15. Which x-ray generator is considered the most efficient at producing x-rays?

_____

16. The standard 60-Hz frequency of an electric current is brought up to what level in a high-frequency x-ray generator?

_____

17. Name four advantages of using high-frequency generators.

_____

_____

18. The most common type of x-ray exposure timer is the:

_____.

19. Which exposure control system requires that the kVp, mA, and exposure time be individually selected?

_____

20. With automatic exposure control, which technical factor is automatically selected?

_____

21. When using automatic exposure control for the exposure, what must be absolutely accurate to ensure that a correct exposure will occur?

_____

22. If overcollimation occurs when using automatic exposure control, the resultant image will be:

_____.

23. If the automatic exposure control system fails for any reason, what system will engage to terminate the exposure?

_____

24. According to Public Law 90-602, x-ray generators must terminate the exposure at what mAs?

_____

25. When using anatomically programmed radiography for the exposure technique, what technical factors are automatically set?

_____

26. The maximum x-ray tube capacity for a single x-ray exposure can be determined by consulting the:

_____.

27. What is the formula for determining a heat unit (HU)?

_____

28. Calculate a heat unit (HU) for an x-ray technique of 300 mA, 65 kVp, 0.10 sec for a (1) single-phase generator; (2) three-phase generator; and (3) high-frequency generator.

    1. _____

    2. _____

    3. _____

29. X-ray tubes will last longer if they are operated at what capacity or less?

_____

30. What can happen to an x-ray tube if it is not warmed up properly?

_____

31. Describe how warm-up x-ray exposures should be made.

_____

32. List five recommendations for prolonging x-ray tube life.

_____

_____

14. Fog affects radiographic quality by causing:
    A. decreased contrast.
    B. underexposure.
    C. increased contrast.
    D. distortion.

15. Motion of the patient, either voluntary or involuntary, during the exposure will result in decreased:
    A. contrast.
    B. distortion.
    C. radiographic density.
    D. detail.

16. A term used to describe a grainy or mottled image is:
    A. umbra.
    B. distortion.
    C. quantum mottle.
    D. penumbra.

17. One means of controlling distortion is by controlling the:
    A. focal spot.
    B. motion.
    C. part position.
    D. quantum mottle.

18. The factors that affect the quantity of x-rays in the x-ray beam are:
    1. mAs.
    2. kVp.
    3. anatomically programmed radiography (APR).
    A. 1 and 2
    B. 1 and 3
    C. 2 and 3
    D. 1, 2, and 3

19. Which of the following will affect the quality of the x-ray beam?
    A. mAs
    B. kVp
    C. anatomically programmed radiography (APR)
    D. automatic exposure control (AEC)

20. If the mAs is doubled, the dose to the patient will:
    A. increase by 10%.
    B. double.
    C. increase by a factor of 4.
    D. remain the same.

21. According to the inverse square law, if the SID is doubled (e.g., 40 inches to 80 inches), the intensity or quantity of x-rays will:
    A. double.
    B. increase by 50%.
    C. be cut in half.
    D. decrease to one-fourth of the original intensity.

22. The principal means of controlling involuntary motion is to:
    A. increase the mA.
    B. increase the kVp.
    C. use a short exposure time.
    D. use a long exposure time.

23. Which one of the following could you use to control spatial resolution?
    A. kVp
    B. Focal spot
    C. Part position
    D. CR angle

24. (True/False) A doubling in kVp would result in four times more x-rays being emitted from the tube.

25. (True/False) If the SID is increased or decreased, the density on the image is not changed.

26. (True/False) If the SID is reduced in half (e.g., 40 inches to 20 inches), the intensity or quantity of x-rays will increase by four times.

27. (True/False) The contrast on the viewing monitor is adjusted by controlling the window level.

28. (True/False) The sharpness in the radiographic image is referred to as spatial resolution.

29. (True/False) Increased quantum mottle will result in increased spatial resolution.

EXERCISE 2

Match the following terms with the corresponding definitions or descriptions.

1. _____ OID

2. _____ Penumbra

3. _____ Inverse square law

4. _____ SID

5. _____ Size distortion

6. _____ Elongation

7. _____ Shape distortion

8. _____ Foreshortening

9. _____ Density

10. _____ Long-scale contrast

11. _____ Contrast

12. _____ Short-scale contrast

13. _____ Quantum mottle

A. Source–image receptor distance

B. Intensity is inversely proportional to the square of the distance

C. Object–image receptor distance

D. Result of unequal magnification

E. Overall blackness on the image

F. Magnification of a part

G. Unsharp edges

H. Difference in density between adjacent structures

I. Object appears shorter

J. Object appears longer

K. Produced by low kVp

L. Produced by high kVp

M. Grainy or mottled image

EXERCISE 3

Answer the following questions.

1. Which of the prime factors of exposure are directly proportional to the quantity of exposure?

   _____

2. What unit is used to indicate the total quantity of exposure?

   _____

3. If an exposure is made using 300 mA, 0.3 sec, 85 kVp, and 40-inch SID, what is the value of the mAs?

   _____

4. If the radiographic image is too dark, which exposure factor(s) would you change to solve the problem?

   _____

5. When the goal is to differentiate between tissues that have very similar densities, is a long or short scale of contrast most desirable? Why?

   _____

   _____

6. What should you do if motion is anticipated in advance of making the exposure?

_____

_____

_____

7. List two possible causes when a radiographic image appears gray and "flat."

    1. _____

    2. _____

8. If a large OID produces an unacceptable loss of spatial resolution, what other factors can be changed to improve the image?

_____

_____

9. When an overall radiographic image appears blurred, what aspect of image quality is affected? Which exposure factor might be changed to solve this problem?

_____

_____

10. List at least three measures that should be taken to prevent voluntary motion during radiography.

    1. _____

    2. _____

    3. _____

11. List at least three factors that will affect radiographic contrast.

    1. _____

    2. _____

    3. _____

12. List the five factors that will affect distortion.

    1. _____

    2. _____

    3. _____

    4. _____

    5. _____

13. List at least five factors that will increase spatial resolution in the radiographic image.

1. _____

2. _____

3. _____

4. _____

5. _____

14. Name the four prime factors of radiographic exposure:

1. _____

2. _____

3. _____

4. _____

15. The digital imaging term for density is: _____.

16. The brightness of the viewing monitor in digital imaging is adjusted by the:

_____.

17. Which photographic factor makes the anatomy in the image visible?

_____

18. What is the name of the tool that is used to simulate different densities on a radiograph?

_____

19. High contrast can also be called:

_____.

20. Low contrast can also be called:

_____.

21. Which two factors affect the subject contrast?

1. _____

2. _____

22. Unwanted exposure in the radiographic image is called:

_____.

Chapter **7** **Principles of Exposure and Image Quality**

20. Define contrast.

_____

21. Define distortion.

_____

22. Define spatial resolution.

_____

23. The term used to describe a dark image is:

_____

24. The term used to describe a light image is:

_____

25. Tissue density refers to:

_____

26. What is the term used to describe density in the digital environment?

_____

27. How does a decrease in kVp affect contrast? An increase in kVp?

_____

28. What is a penetrometer?

_____

29. Describe short-scale contrast and long-scale contrast.

_____

30. The densities of the tissues within the patient are referred to as:

_____

31. Contrast is influenced by:

_____

32. Describe the term *fog.*

_____

33. How does collimation affect fog?

_____

34. What term is used to describe contrast in the digital environment?

_____

35. Low kVp produces an image with what type of contrast?

_____

36. High kVp produces an image with what type of contrast?

_____

37. Another name for size distortion is:

_____

38. The distance between the body part and the IR is called the:

_____

39. Define elongation.

_____

40. Define foreshortening.

_____

41. What are the five factors that affect spatial resolution?

_____

_____

42. Having unsharp or fuzzy edges of structures in an image is called:

_____

43. Changing from the small to the large focal spot results in:

_____

44. An increase in the OID will result in:

_____

45. Motion of the patient, tube, or IR during the exposure results in:

_____

46. If an x-ray image is blurred or has motion, which exposure factors are used to correct this?

_____

47. Patient motion can be categorized in what two ways?

_____

48. The first step in avoiding motion is to use:

_____.

49. The principal method of reducing involuntary motion is to:

_____.

50. The technical term for a grainy or spotty image is:

_____.

51. What causes an image to have a grainy appearance?

_____

52. What are two ways to minimize shape distortion?

_____

53. Name three things that will increase spatial resolution.

_____

_____

8 | Digital Imaging

EXERCISE 1

Match the following terms with their descriptions.

1. _____ Digital imaging

2. _____ Computed radiography (CR)

3. _____ Photostimulable storage phosphor (PSP)

4. _____ Digital radiography (DR)

5. _____ Indirect conversion

6. _____ Direct conversion

7. _____ Postprocessing

A. A "cassette-less" digital x-ray system

B. A "cassette-based" digital x-ray system

C. Means for adjusting any image of a body part with computer software

D. Process in which detectors convert x-ray energy directly into an electrical signal

E. General term for the process of acquiring images of the body using x-rays, displaying them digitally, and viewing and storing them on computers

F. Two-step process in which x-ray energy is converted to light and then to an electrical signal

G. Stores the image of the body part

EXERCISE 2

Match the following terms with their descriptions.

1. _____ Brightness

2. _____ Contrast resolution

3. _____ Quantum mottle

4. _____ Matrix

5. _____ Pixel

6. _____ Spatial resolution

7. _____ Window level

8. _____ Window width

A. Describes x-ray images that are grainy or mottled (spotty), caused when not enough photons reach the detector

B. Ability to distinguish anatomic structures of similar subject contrast

C. A control that adjusts the density in the image

D. A series of thousands of small squares that make up the viewing monitor's active area

E. A control that adjusts the contrast in the image

F. The amount of detail or sharpness of an image as seen on the viewing monitor

G. Used in place of "density" in digital imaging

H. An individual square or picture element in the monitor's active area

EXERCISE 3

Answer the following questions by selecting the best choice.

1. Which of the following modalities in radiology produces digital images that can be sent through a computer network?
   1. Computed tomography
   2. Magnetic resonance imaging
   3. Conventional radiography
   A. 1 and 2
   B. 1 and 3
   C. 2 and 3
   D. 1, 2, and 3

2. Which of the following is used in computed radiography (CR) to store a digital image?
   A. Laser light
   B. PSP plate
   C. Flat-panel detector
   D. Film or screen cassette

3. The phosphor used in the CR imaging plate is:
   A. lanthanum.
   B. gadolinium.
   C. yttrium.
   D. barium fluorohalide with europium.

4. Which of the following is/are necessary to process a CR image?
   1. Darkroom
   2. CR reader unit
   3. Computer systems with monitors
   A. 1 and 2
   B. 1 and 3
   C. 2 and 3
   D. 1, 2, and 3

5. After an imaging plate is scanned by the CR reader unit, it is erased with:
   A. laser light.
   B. white light.
   C. red light.
   D. fluorescent light.

6. One of the most important aspects of setting the exposure technique when using digital imaging systems is to ensure that which of the following is correctly set on the generator?
   A. kVp
   B. SID
   C. mA
   D. Exposure time

7. Which of the following is a true statement regarding the use of collimation with digital systems?
   A. At least two sides of collimation should be seen on the image.
   B. No collimation edges should be seen on the image.
   C. At least 1 cm of collimation should be seen on all four sides.
   D. At least 2 cm of collimation should be seen on two of the sides.

8. The erasure process will begin if a CR cassette is opened and the plate is exposed for:
   A. 5 sec.
   B. 10 sec.
   C. 15 sec.
   D. 20 sec.

9. The photoconductor used in digital radiography (DR) flat-panel detectors is:
   A. amorphous selenium and silicon.
   B. barium fluorohalide.
   C. solidified copper.
   D. carbon fiber.

10. A major advantage of CR and DR digital imaging systems is:
    A. elimination of repeat images.
    B. higher-contrast images.
    C. the ability to see images very fast.
    D. a lower dose to the patient.

11. The viewing monitor's active area is made up of thousands of small squares called the:
    A. flat panel.
    B. dynamic range.
    C. pixels.
    D. matrix.

12. How many pixels are there in a 1650 × 1800 viewing monitor?
    A. 2500
    B. 2900
    C. 2,500,000
    D. 2,970,000

13. Which matrix below will provide the greatest spatial resolution?
    A. 800 × 1200
    B. 1650 × 1800
    C. 1800 × 2250
    D. 2000 × 2500

14. The response of the detector to different levels of radiation exposure is termed:
    A. spatial resolution.
    B. the dynamic range.
    C. shuttering.
    D. the signal-to-noise ratio.

15. The ability of a digital system to convert the x-ray input electrical signal into a useful radiographic image is termed the:
    A. contrast resolution.
    B. spatial resolution.
    C. dynamic range.
    D. signal-to-noise ratio.

16. With direct-conversion DR, the x-ray energy is directly converted to:
    A. light.
    B. light and then an electrical signal.
    C. an electrical signal.
    D. an electrical signal and then a capacitor.

17. Which of the following takes the stored charge in the flat-panel detector and converts it into digital value?
    A. Charged coupled device (CCD)
    B. Analog-to-digital converter (ADC)
    C. Complementary metal oxide semiconductor (CMOS)
    D. Smoothing processor

18. The universally accepted standard for exchanging medical images is termed:
    A. DICOM.
    B. PACS.
    C. SNL.
    D. ALARA.

19. The image management system used in a digital radiology department is called:
    A. PSP.
    B. SNL.
    C. PACS.
    D. DICOM.

20. When using a CR plate, how much of the energy of the latent image is lost if the plate is not processed within 8 hours?
    A. 5%
    B. 10%
    C. 15%
    D. 25%

21. Which of the following will be seen in the x-ray image if either the kVp or the mA is set to low for the projection?
    A. Quantum mottle.
    B. Low-contrast resolution.
    C. Greater brightness.
    D. High signal-to-noise ratio.

22. What is the name of the processing technique in which x-ray images can be made sharper and have greatly increased contrast?
    A. Smoothing.
    B. Edge enhancement.
    C. Shuttering.
    D. Rescaling.

EXERCISE 4

Fill in the blanks with the correct word or words.

1. With CR digital systems, the imaging plate is scanned with a(n) _____ after being inserted into the reader device.

2. The phosphor plate inside the CR cassette can be used _____ times before it needs to be replaced.

3. The phosphor that absorbs the x-ray energy in a(n) _____ system is called a *flat-panel detector.*

4. Name at least two major advantages of using CR and DR systems.

    1. _____

    2. _____

5. _____ will occur in digital systems if there are too few photons reaching the IR.

6. In DR environments, the abbreviation *PACS* stands for _____

_____.

7. _____ should be used for body parts that have extreme differences in tissue density.

8. Because of the wider dynamic range of digital systems, a *slightly* higher _____ setting may be acceptable for radiography projections done using a grid or Bucky.

9. If a CR plate is divided in half and used for two separate exposures, the side not receiving the exposure must always

be _____.

10. The storage phosphors in CR plates are hypersensitive to _____.

11. With CR and DR, images can be processed and seen in _____ seconds.

12. In digital imaging, unwanted graininess in the image is called _____.

13. With DR indirect conversion, _____ steps are required to process the image.

14. Two postprocessing techniques are:

    1. _____

    2. _____

15. The method for calibrating a particular display system for the purpose of presenting images consistently on different viewing monitors and printers is called the:

_____.

16. Name at least six artifact patterns seen in digital imaging.

    1. _____

    2. _____

    3. _____

    4. _____

    5. _____

    6. _____

17. The technique that can be useful in viewing very small structures and the fine details of bone is called

_____.

18. When the x-ray exposure is greater or less than what is needed to produce an image, automatic _____ occurs.

EXERCISE 5

Fill in the blanks with T or F to indicate whether each of the following statements is true or false.

1. _____ An exposure technique chart is not necessary when using digital imaging systems.

2. _____ With direct-conversion DR, the x-ray energy is converted directly into an electrical signal.

3. _____ Subtraction and contrast enhancement are postprocessing techniques.

4. _____ CR imaging plates should never be split to enable two separate exposures on one plate.

5. _____ CR imaging plates are more sensitive to scatter radiation both before and after exposure to x-rays.

6. _____ When there is a high signal-to-noise ratio, the least amount of information is captured.

EXERCISE 6

Match the following terms with their descriptions.

1. _____ Analog-to-digital converter (ADC)

2. _____ Dead pixels

3. _____ Rescaling

4. _____ Smoothing

5. _____ Edge enhancement

6. _____ Dynamic range

A. A processing technique in which each pixel's frequency is averaged with the surrounding tissue's pixel values. This is done to remove noise, which can be bothersome to the radiologist.

B. Takes the stored charge from the detector and converts it into a digital value.

C. When the x-ray exposure is greater or less than what is needed to produce an image, this processing system is engaged. It is designed to display all the pixels for the area of interest with uniform density and contrast.

D. The response of the detector to different levels of radiation exposure.

E. Occurs when there may be a defect in a component of the computer screen matrix. This may cause a loss of patient information.

F. A processing technique in which images can be made sharper and have greatly increased contrast; however, it does introduce some noise and loss of detail.

CHALLENGE EXERCISE

This exercise does not have to be completed at the same time as the other exercises in this workbook chapter. The exercise is designed to assess retention of the essential information contained in the corresponding textbook chapter. It is recommended that you complete this exercise when you begin to study for the state limited licensure examination. This will help determine what you know and which information should be further reviewed.

1. What is the name of the cassette-based digital imaging system?

_____

2. The PSP in the CR imaging plate is:

_____.

3. Imaging plates from digital CR are processed in a(n):

_____.

4. How many times can a CR imaging plate be used?

_____

5. How does scatter radiation affect the CR imaging plate?

_____

6. What type of light source is used in the CR reader unit to release the stored x-ray energy?

_____

7. What type of light source is used to erase the stored image in a CR imaging plate?

_____

8. The cassette-less digital imaging system is called:

_____

9. A flat-panel detector is used in which digital imaging system?

_____

10. What material is used as the conductor in a direct conversion flat-panel detector system?

_____

11. What is the size of the flat-panel detector in the table of a DR imaging system?

_____

12. What are the two categories of DR imaging systems?

    1. _____

    2. _____

13. How long does it take to process a CR or DR image using a general digital system?

_____

14. One of the major advantages of digital imaging systems is the ability to:

_____.

15. What are the two steps in processing an indirect-conversion DR image?

    1. _____

    2. _____

16. With direct-conversion DR systems, the x-ray energy is converted directly to:

_____.

17. On a digital viewing monitor, the active area of the monitor is called the:

_____.

18. On a digital viewing monitor, each individual picture element square is called a(n):

_____.

19. The amount of detail or sharpness in a digital image is termed:

_____.

20. How many pixels are there in a 1200 × 1200–matrix viewing monitor?

_____

21. How do smaller pixels affect spatial resolution?

_____

22. How will a larger matrix affect the pixels?

_____

23. The ability of a digital system to distinguish anatomic structures that have a similar subject contrast is termed:

_____.

24. The number of gray shades that an imaging system can produce is termed:

_____.

25. "Noise" in the digital image is referred to as:

_____.

26. The ability of a digital system to convert the x-ray–input electrical signal into a useful image is termed:

_____.

27. How does a greater electrical signal in a digital imaging system affect noise and image quality?

_____

28. What adjustment controls the density or brightness of the digital image on the viewing monitor and printed image?

_____

29. What adjustment controls the contrast of the digital image on the viewing monitor and printed image?

_____

30. What two entities require that exposure technique charts be placed in every radiography room?

　　1. _____

　　2. _____

31. The acronym for maintaining optimal image quality and low radiation exposure to the patient is:

　　_____.

32. One of the most important aspects of setting the exposure technique in digital imaging systems is to ensure that which factor is set correctly?

　　_____

33. What is the name of the device that takes the stored charge in the detector and converts it into digital values?

　　_____

34. What are the names of the two types of indirect conversion flat-panel detectors?

　　_____

35. The further adjustment of a digital image after it is processed is termed:

　　_____.

36. The universally accepted standard for exchanging medical images and viewing images from different manufacturers is termed:

　　_____.

37. The method of calibrating a digital display system so that all images are presented consistently is termed:

　　_____.

38. Two common postprocessing techniques are:

　　_____.

39. What causes the quantum mottle artifact in the digital image?

　　_____

40. What causes the moiré pattern artifact in the digital image?

　　_____

41. What causes the phantom or ghost image artifact in the digital image?

　　_____

42. What causes the fogged image artifact in the digital image?

_____

43. What causes extraneous line pattern artifacts in the digital image?

_____

44. The management system used in digital imaging to store and view images is termed:

_____.

45. What types of patient information must be included on every digital image?

_____

46. What technical exposure adjustment can be made to reduce radiation exposure to the patient?

_____

47. What device should be used when imaging body parts that have widely different thicknesses of structures?

_____

48. What types of images from a radiology department are stored in a PACS system?

_____

49. Where should the body part be ideally placed on a CR plate?

_____

50. What device should be available if one CR plate is divided in half for two images?

_____

51. If a digital image appears on the viewing monitor as overexposed or underexposed, what should be checked?

_____

52. How many margins of the collimator should ideally be seen on a digital image?

_____

53. With CR imaging plates, how much of the energy of the x-ray image in the phosphor is lost in 8 hours?

_____

54. Defective pixels are caused by:

_____.

55. What is the name of the processing technique in which images can be made sharper and have greatly increased contrast?

_____

56. What is the name of the technique in which each pixel's frequency is averaged with the surrounding tissue's pixel values in an effort to reduce noise in the image?

_____

57. What is the name of the processing technique that allows x-ray images to be produced with uniform density and contrast, regardless of the amount of exposure?

_____

9 Scatter Radiation and Its Control

EXERCISE 1

Answer the following questions by selecting the best choice.

1. Radiation produced by the photoelectric effect is called:
   A. scattered radiation.
   B. the Compton effect.
   C. secondary radiation.
   D. coherent scattering.

2. Scattered radiation affects the radiographic image by causing:
   1. fog.
   2. reduced contrast.
   3. reduced recorded detail.
   A. 1 and 2
   B. 1 and 3
   C. 2 and 3
   D. 1, 2, and 3

3. Which of the following factors will affect the quantity of scattered radiation fog on a radiograph?
   1. Peak kilovoltage (kVp)
   2. Computed radiography (CR) plate
   3. Field size
   A. 1 and 2
   B. 1 and 3
   C. 2 and 3
   D. 1, 2, and 3

4. The most effective method of reducing scattered radiation fog on a radiograph is to:
   A. decrease the object–image receptor distance (OID).
   B. decrease the source–image receptor distance (SID).
   C. increase the kVp.
   D. use a grid or Bucky.

5. As the kVp is increased, the photoelectric effect:
   A. is decreased.
   B. is increased.
   C. remains the same.
   D. remains the same if the kVp is less than 60.

6. As the kVp is increased, the Compton effect:
   A. is decreased.
   B. is increased.
   C. remains the same.
   D. remains the same if the kVp is less than 60.

7. On a radiograph, the appearance of decreased density on the side of the image is most likely caused by the:
   A. grid motion.
   B. grid cutoff.
   C. grid ratio.
   D. grid frequency.

8. A moving grid may be part of a radiographic table or upright unit and is called a:
   A. Bucky grid.
   B. cross-hatch grid.
   C. focused grid.
   D. linear grid.

9. What effect does a thicker or larger body part have on scatter radiation?
   A. There will be greater scatter.
   B. There will be less scatter.
   C. Scatter will remain the same.
   D. Scatter can increase or decrease depending on the atomic number of the part.

10. The central ray alignment quality control test must show that the alignment is within _____ degree(s) of perpendicular.
   A. 1
   B. 2
   C. 3
   D. 4

11. When a body part is dense, or has a greater atomic number, scatter radiation:
   A. is increased.
   B. is decreased.
   C. remains the same.
   D. remains the same if the kVp is greater than 60.

12. Which of the following will reduce scatter radiation?
   A. Increase the kVp.
   B. Use a smaller field size.
   C. Increase the SID.
   D. Decrease the milliampere-seconds (mAs).

13. In the diagnostic range of kVp settings (50 to 100 kVp), the majority of scattered radiation will be from which interaction with matter?
   A. Compton effect
   B. Coherent scattering
   C. Photoelectric effect
   D. Characteristic radiation

14. Total absorption of an x-ray photon by the atom of the body part is termed:
    A. the Compton effect.
    B. coherent scattering.
    C. the photoelectric effect.
    D. characteristic radiation.

15. The majority of photons that are scattered will scatter in which direction?
    A. Toward the head
    B. Toward the feet
    C. Back toward the x-ray tube
    D. In a more forward direction

16. The control limit for the collimator on the x-ray tube is that it must be maintained within a range of:
    A. ±2% of the SID.
    B. ±3% of the SID.
    C. ±4% of the SID.
    D. ±5% of the SID.

17. The principal source of scatter radiation is the:
    A. tabletop.
    B. patient.
    C. grid.
    D. image receptor.

18. A grid is used when the body part becomes larger than:
    A. 5 cm.
    B. 8 cm.
    C. 10 to 12 cm.
    D. 12 to 14 cm.

EXERCISE 2

Fill in the blanks with T or F to indicate whether each of the following statements is true or false.

1. _____ Higher kVp results in more scattered radiation fog.

2. _____ The quality control test of the collimator field and x-ray field must show that the two fields are within 2% of the SID.

3. _____ As the kVp is increased, the Compton effect is decreased.

4. _____ As the kVp is increased, the photoelectric effect is increased.

5. _____ The production of scatter results in fog on the radiograph.

6. _____ As collimation is increased, or made larger, scatter radiation fog is decreased.

7. _____ The atomic number of the body part influences the quantity of scatter radiation fog.

8. _____ ↑ *Tissue thickness* = ↑ interactions = ↑ scatter = ↑ fog.

9. _____ The patient is the principal source of scattered radiation in radiography.

10. _____ A grid is placed between the patient and the image receptor (IR).

11. _____ Compton scatter travels in a forward direction only.

12. _____ Scatter radiation fog reduces the visibility of detail.

13. _____ The standard control limit for the x-ray tube's central ray alignment is that the tube must be mounted so that the beam is within 1 degree of perpendicular.

14. _____ The collimator and the beam alignment must be checked using two separate quality control tests.

EXERCISE 3

Answer the following questions.

1. Which type of radiation interaction produces scattered radiation that is characteristic of the subject irradiated?

   _____

   _____

2. List the two factors that affect the volume of tissue irradiated.

   1. _____

   2. _____

3. When the kVp is increased, will the quantity of secondary radiation fog be increased or decreased? Why?

   _____

   _____

4. What is the principal source of scattered radiation that causes fog in radiography?

   _____

   _____

5. State the four factors that directly affect the quantity of scatter radiation fog.

   1. _____

   2. _____

   3. _____

   4. _____

6. The *primary* scatter consideration is the:

   _____

7. Why is there less scatter radiation with a body part that is more dense or has a higher atomic number?

   _____

8. One of the most important things a limited operator can do to control scatter radiation is to:

   _____

9. What are the names of the two test tools used to perform a quality control check of the collimator and the central ray alignment?

1. _____

2. _____

10. What happens to the x-ray photon when the Compton effect is occurring?

_____

11. What happens to the x-ray photon during the photoelectric effect?

_____

CHALLENGE EXERCISE

This exercise does not have to be completed at the same time as the other exercises in this workbook chapter. The exercise is designed to assess retention of the essential information contained in the corresponding textbook chapter. It is recommended that you complete this exercise when you begin to study for the state limited licensure examination. This will help determine what you know and which information should be further reviewed.

1. The two main types of interactions that occur when radiation is absorbed by matter are:

1. _____

2. _____

2. Compton scatter leaves the body in what directions?

_____

3. Scatter radiation that is directed back toward the x-ray tube is termed:

_____

4. Most of the photons that scatter will scatter in which specific direction?

_____

5. What happens to the x-ray photon during the Compton effect?

_____

6. What happens to the x-ray photon during the photoelectric effect?

_____

7. What happens to the energy of the photon when it is scattered?

_____

8. When the kVp is increased, the Compton scatter is:

_____

9. When the kVp is increased, the photoelectric effect is:

   _____.

10. The production of scatter radiation during an exposure results in what effect on the x-ray image?

    _____

11. Name the four primary factors that directly affect the quantity of scatter radiation fog:

    1. _____

    2. _____

    3. _____

    4. _____

12. The primary consideration that affects the volume of scatter radiation is the:

    _____.

13. How is scatter affected when the body part is thicker or larger?

    _____

14. Fog on the radiograph becomes objectionable when the body part size is larger than:

    _____.

15. What is the effect of increased kVp on scatter radiation fog?

    _____

16. How is scatter affected when a body part is very dense or has a high atomic number?

    _____

17. One of the most important things a limited operator can do to control scatter radiation is:

    _____.

18. The principal method of reducing scatter radiation fog is to use which device?

    _____

19. Name three strategies that can be used to reduce scatter radiation fog.

    1. _____

    2. _____

    3. _____

20. A grid is typically used when the body part size and kVp reach:

_____.

21. What does decreasing collimation do to the contrast in the image?

_____

22. When fog prevents specific details from being seen in the image, what type of image may be requested?

_____

23. Name the two quality control tests that are done regularly to check the collimator's light field size and the central ray alignment.

　　1. _____

　　2. _____

24. Name the test tools used to check the collimator's light field and also the central ray alignment.

　　1. _____

　　2. _____

25. The control limit for the collimator's light field and the actual radiation field must be within:

_____.

26. The control limit for the x-ray tube's beam alignment is that the beam must be within:

_____.

10 Formulating X-ray Techniques

EXERCISE 1

Answer the following questions by selecting the best choice.

1. A technique chart provides the following information:
   1. Milliamperage (mA).
   2. Peak kilovoltage (kVp).
   3. Source–image receptor distance (SID).
   A. 1 and 2
   B. 1 and 3
   C. 2 and 3
   D. 1, 2, and 3

2. Which of the following methods is an effective way to obtain a technique chart?
   1. Have each x-ray operator write down the techniques for 1 week.
   2. Request assistance from the imaging manufacturer's technical representative.
   3. Hire a consultant who is an expert in technique chart preparation.
   A. 1 and 2
   B. 1 and 3
   C. 2 and 3
   D. 1, 2, and 3

3. Manual technique charts are based on patient part measurements obtained using an x-ray caliper. These measurements are expressed as:
   A. depth, in inches.
   B. circumference, in inches.
   C. thickness, in centimeters.
   D. diameter, in millimeters.

4. The kVp that is sufficient to penetrate the body part adequately without excess exposure to the patient is called:
   A. fixed kVp.
   B. optimum kVp.
   C. variable kVp.
   D. manual kVp.

5. What factors need to be considered when selecting the mA station?
   1. Exposure time
   2. Focal spot size
   3. Thickness of the patient part
   A. 1 and 2
   B. 1 and 3
   C. 2 and 3
   D. 1, 2, and 3

6. When selecting a low mA station (100 mA), you should use:
   A. the large focal spot.
   B. the small focal spot.
   C. either the large or small focal spot.

7. The advantages of using a variable kVp technique chart are:
   1. lower image contrast.
   2. improved visibility of detail.
   3. the ability to make small incremental changes in exposure technique.
   A. 1 and 2
   B. 1 and 3
   C. 2 and 3
   D. 1, 2, and 3

8. Why should the small focal spot be used as much as possible?
   A. It provides better image sharpness.
   B. It provides better contrast.
   C. It reduces anode heat.
   D. It reduces patient motion.

9. How should exposure factors be adjusted when there is the likelihood of motion?
   A. ↑ mA, ↓ exposure time
   B. ↓ mA, ↑ exposure time
   C. ↓ mA, ↓ exposure time
   D. ↑ mA, ↑ exposure time

10. A satisfactory radiograph is made using 5 milliampere-seconds (mAs) with an image receptor relative speed (RS) of 400. How many mAs would be necessary to produce a radiograph of similar density if an RS 100 screen were used?
    A. 1.25 mAs
    B. 10 mAs
    C. 15 mAs
    D. 20 mAs

11. Which mA station can be used for most average-size patients to take advantage of the small focal spot?
    A. 50
    B. 100
    C. 200
    D. 400

12. The official organization that accredits hospitals and clinics and requires technique charts is:
    A. The Joint Commission.
    B. the American Registry of Radiologic Technologists.
    C. the American Society of Radiologic Technologists.
    D. the State Hospital Association.

13. One advantage of using a fixed exposure technique chart is that:
    A. the contrast will be increased for all images.
    B. the exposures will have more latitude for exposure error.
    C. the dose to the patient will be reduced.
    D. fewer repeat exposures are performed.

14. By how much do the mAs have to be changed to see a visible shift in image density?
    A. 5%
    B. 10%
    C. 25%
    D. 30%

15. Which of the following x-ray projections can benefit from the use of compensating filters?
    A. Anteroposterior (AP) thoracic spine
    B. Axiolateral hip
    C. AP skull
    D. Both A and B

16. (True/False) Once established on the technique chart, the kVp should never be changed unless the contrast needs to be changed.

17. (True/False) If a compensating filter is used with a body part that has significantly varying tissue density, such as the shoulder in an AP projection, two separate exposures will still have to be made.

18. (True/False) The use of compensating filters can help reduce the entrance skin exposure.

19. (True/False) The major limitation in obtaining images of obese patients is inadequate penetration of the body part.

20. (True/False) The most important adjustment that can be made on an obese patient is the mA.

EXERCISE 2

Indicate the correct mAs for the new source–image receptor distance (SID) to maintain density.

1. If 25 mAs at 40 inches, calculate the mAs at 80 inches.

2. If 30 mAs at 60 inches, calculate the mAs at 30 inches.

EXERCISE 3

Label the following with an up arrow (↑) to indicate the need for increased technique or a down arrow (↓) to indicate the need for decreased technique.

1. _____ Paget's disease

2. _____ Edema

3. _____ Bowel obstruction

4. _____ Sarcoma

5. _____ Hemothorax

6. _____ Pneumothorax

7. _____ Bronchiectasis

8. _____ Advanced age

9. _____ Degenerative arthritis

10. _____ Gout

11. _____ Atelectasis

12. _____ Chronic obstructive pulmonary disease (COPD)

13. _____ Metastases

14. _____ Pleural effusion

EXERCISE 4

Answer the following questions.

1. Using the technique chart from your facility or the one provided in Appendix D in your textbook, state the exposure factors for a lateral chest radiograph on a patient measuring 32 cm.

   _____

   _____

2. Which tool and which units are used to measure body part thickness for radiography?

   _____

   _____

3. The mA should be kept below what level in order to use the small focal spot and obtain better detail?

   _____

4. Using the table of optimum kVp ranges in Appendix E in your textbook, state the optimum kVp ranges for AP projections of the cervical spine, thoracic spine, and lumbar spine.

   _____

   _____

   _____

5. Assume that your x-ray control panel has the following mA settings: 50, 100, 200, and 300. Which might you use for radiography of the elbow? The lumbar spine? The chest?

   _____

   _____

_____

_____

6. You are about to take a radiograph that requires 10 mAs, and you have decided to use 100 mA. What should the exposure time setting be?

_____

7. List two pathologic conditions that require an exposure increase and two that require a decrease.

Increase:

1. _____

2. _____

Decrease:

1. _____

2. _____

8. An acceptable radiograph is made using 200 mA, 0.3 sec, and 70 kVp. Calculate a new exposure that will provide more latitude (lower contrast) and less patient dose for the same examination on the same patient.

_____

_____

_____

_____

9. If a satisfactory radiograph is made using 20 mAs at 40 inches of SID, how many mAs would be necessary to produce a similar radiograph at 72 inches of SID?

_____

_____

_____

10. Name three reasons why an exposure technique chart may not work properly.

1. _____

2. _____

3. _____

11. A general rule of thumb for mAs changes when an image is too light or too dark is to make adjustments in increments of:

_____

12. When using the 15% rule, a 15% change in kVp will produce approximately the same changes in radiographic density as:

_____.

CHALLENGE EXERCISE

This exercise does not have to be completed at the same time as the other exercises in this workbook chapter. The exercise is designed to assess retention of the essential information contained in the corresponding textbook chapter. It is recommended that you complete this exercise when you begin to study for the state limited licensure examination. This will help determine what you know and which information should be further reviewed.

1. A listing of the examinations and the exposure factors used for those examinations that must be placed in every room is called the:

_____.

2. What is the name of the organization that provides accreditation for hospitals and clinics?

_____

3. Name several technical factors that must be included on an exposure technique chart.

_____

_____

4. A technique chart that requires every factor to be set individually is called a(n):

_____.

5. An exposure technique chart may not need to be posted for the _____ type of exposure control system.

6. What is the name of the device or tool used to measure patient part size?

_____

7. The kVp can be determined for a technique chart using what two types of kVp settings?

    1. _____

    2. _____

8. What does "optimal kVp" mean?

_____

9. What does the "15% rule" mean?

_____

10. The small focal spot can only be used at which mA settings?

_____

11. When there is a likelihood of motion in a radiograph, how should the mA and exposure time be set?

_____

12. Name two ways in which an exposure technique chart can fail.

1. _____

2. _____

13. Name at least six pathologic conditions that would require an *increase* in exposure factors.

1. _____

2. _____

3. _____

4. _____

5. _____

6. _____

14. Name at least six pathologic conditions that would require a *decrease* in exposure factors.

1. _____

2. _____

3. _____

4. _____

5. _____

6. _____

15. Specialty exposure technique charts must be provided for which two diverse groups of patients?

1. _____

2. _____

16. The major limitation in imaging obese patients is:

_____.

17. What is the most important technical factor adjustment that should be made when imaging obese patients?

_____

18. What is the minimum change in mAs that will prompt a visible change in image density?

_____

19. When a radiograph needs to be repeated because the original image was too dark or too light, what is the minimum change in mAs that should be made in each case?

_____

20. What is the formula used if the mAs has to be adjusted because of a change in SID?

_____

21. What type of body part will require a compensating filter?

_____

22. Name at least four body parts or x-ray projections for which a compensating filter will help obtain a radiograph of more even density.

1. _____

2. _____

3. _____

4. _____

23. Where are compensating filters placed?

_____

11 Radiobiology and Radiation Safety

Answer the following questions by selecting the best choice.

1. The International System of Units (SI) unit for measuring the *absorbed dose* in the patient is the:
   A. roentgen (R).
   B. gray-$_t$ (Gy-$_t$).
   C. gray-$_a$ (Gy-$_a$).
   D. sievert (Sv).

2. The SI measurement of radiation *exposure* in air is the:
   A. roentgen (R).
   B. gray-$_t$ (Gy-$_t$).
   C. gray-$_a$ (Gy-$_a$).
   D. sievert (Sv).

3. The SI unit used to report the *equivalent dose,* or occupational dose, to radiation workers in the United States is the:
   A. roentgen (R).
   B. gray-$_t$ (Gy-$_t$).
   C. gray-$_a$ (Gy-$_a$).
   D. sievert (Sv).

4. According to the law of Bergonié–Tribondeau, which of the following types of cells would be most radiosensitive?
   A. Skin cells
   B. Nerve and muscle cells
   C. Embryonic tissue
   D. Cortical bone

5. *Short-term* effects of radiation are typically observed within:
   A. 1 day.
   B. 3 days.
   C. 1 month.
   D. 3 months.

6. Which of the following is considered an observable *short-term* effect of radiation exposure?
   A. Cataractogenesis
   B. Carcinogenesis
   C. Mutations
   D. Erythema

7. The reduction of a limited operator's exposure to ionizing radiation can be accomplished by:
   1. decreasing the time in the radiation field.
   2. increasing the distance from the radiation source.
   3. using exposure techniques with a low peak kilovoltage (kVp).
   A. 1 and 2
   B. 1 and 3
   C. 2 and 3
   D. 1, 2, and 3

8. The *e* annual *effective dose* limit for a whole-body dose of occupational radiation for nonpregnant workers over the age of 18 is:
   A. 50 millisieverts (mSv).
   B. 500 mSv.
   C. 50 mGy-$_a$.
   D. 500 mGy-$_a$.

9. Which of the following are considered low-dose techniques?
   1. Increasing kVp, decreasing milliampere-seconds (mAs)
   2. Using low milliampere (mA) settings
   3. Using a minimum source–image receptor distance (SID) of 40 inches
   A. 1 and 2
   B. 1 and 3
   C. 2 and 3
   D. 1, 2, and 3

10. Which of the following changes will decrease the patient dose?
    A. Using low-mA settings
    B. Decreasing the filtration
    C. Using high-kVp techniques
    D. Using a 36-inch SID

11. When radiation exposure occurs during pregnancy, the greatest risk of birth defects occurs when the dose to the uterus exceeds:
    A. 5 milligray-$_t$ (mGy-$_t$).
    B. 10 mGy-$_t$.
    C. 15 mGy-$_t$.
    D. 150 mGy-$_t$.

12. Limited operators can reduce radiation risk to their patients by:
    1. minimizing repeat exposures.
    2. using low-kVp techniques.
    3. collimating closely to the part.
    A. 1 and 2
    B. 1 and 3
    C. 2 and 3
    D. 1, 2, and 3

13. The radiation *weighting factor* for x-ray photons is:
    A. 1.
    B. 2.
    C. 3.
    D. 5.

14. An *equivalent dose* of 0.400 Sv would be converted to _____ mSv.
    A. 4.0
    B. 40
    C. 400
    D. 4000

15. In our everyday work, the *equivalent dose* is used for:
    A. air radiation measurements.
    B. measurements of the x-ray room.
    C. radiation protection purposes.
    D. pregnant occupational workers.

16. The greatest cause of unnecessary radiation exposure to patients that can be controlled by the limited operator is:
    A. motion.
    B. repeat exposures.
    C. use of high-kVp techniques.
    D. use of high-mA techniques.

17. Whenever the gonads are within _____ of the margin of the radiation field, gonadal dose will be significantly reduced by shielding.
    A. 2 cm
    B. 4 cm
    C. 5 cm
    D. 6 cm

18. A pregnant radiation worker's monthly *equivalent dose* limit is:
    A. 0.3 mSv.
    B. 0.5 mSv.
    C. 1.0 mSv.
    D. 1.5 mSv.

19. A 33-year-old radiation worker would have a *cumulative effective dose* limit of:
    A. 3 mSv.
    B. 30 mSv.
    C. 33 mSv.
    D. 330 mSv.

20. An *erythema* can develop on a patient if the radiation dose to the skin reaches:
    A. 100 mSv.
    B. 1000 mSv.
    C. 2000 mSv.
    D. 2500 mSv.

21. When the dose to the patient is clarified by the *type and energy* of the radiation, it is termed the:
    A. exposure.
    B. absorbed dose.
    C. equivalent dose.
    D. effective dose.

22. Patient dose in radiography is most often calculated according to the exposure level at the:
    A. skin.
    B. gonads.
    C. collar.
    D. exit of the body part.

23. *Short-term* effects of radiation will occur at doses greater than:
    A. 50 mGy-$_t$.
    B. 100 mGy-$_t$.
    C. 250 mGy-$_t$.
    D. 500 mGy-$_t$.

24. In diagnostic radiology, we are most concerned about which effect of radiation exposure?
    A. Somatic effect
    B. Genetic effect
    C. Long-term effect
    D. Short-term effect

25. The LD 50/30, or the lethal dose that would be fatal to 50% of the irradiated population within 30 days, is:
    A. 3000 mGy-$_t$.
    B. 4000 mGy-$_t$.
    C. 5000 mGy-$_t$.
    D. 5000 to 7000 mGy-$_t$.

26. The greatest percentage of *long-term* effects from radiation exposure will occur:
    A. at 5 years.
    B. at 10 years.
    C. at between 10 and 15 years.
    D. at between 12 and 20 years.

27. Which of the following would be considered a *long-term* effect of radiation exposure?
    1. Cataracts
    2. Life span shortening
    3. Leukemia
    A. 1 and 2
    B. 1 and 3
    C. 2 and 3
    D. 1, 2, and 3

28. (True/False) The standard lead equivalency of the lead aprons used in the radiology department should be a minimum of 0.75-mm lead.

29. (True/False) Radiographers should perform lead apron and glove inspection every 6 months.

30. (True/False) A human who receives an acute whole-body exposure of 6.0 Sv will die.

31. (True/False) The earliest biologic effect that will be seen in the human body after exposure to radiation is nausea and vomiting.

32. (True/False) In diagnostic radiology, the absorbed dose and the equivalent dose are always the same value.

33. (True/False) Younger cells are no more sensitive to radiation than adult cells.

34. (True/False) Long-term effects from radiation exposure are not predictable.

35. (True/False) The greatest risk to a fetus is during the last 3 months of pregnancy.

EXERCISE 2

Match the following terms with their definitions or descriptions.

1. _____ Effective dose

2. _____ Gray-$_t$

3. _____ Long-term somatic

4. _____ Air kerma

5. _____ Equivalent dose

6. _____ Carcinogenesis

7. _____ ALARA

8. _____ Mutation

9. _____ Gonad shield

10. _____ Erythema

11. _____ Entrance skin exposure

A. Radiation burn

B. Upper limit of occupational exposure permissible

C. Genetic changes or effects

D. Device to prevent unnecessary radiation to reproductive organs

E. An effect that is not predictable

F. SI unit used to measure absorbed dose

G. Term used to describe absorbed dose based on type and energy of x-ray

H. SI unit of radiation exposure

I. Radiation exposure should be limited to the lowest possible levels

J. Development of malignant disease

K. Exposure at the skin level

EXERCISE 3

Answer the following questions.

1. Name at least four methods that limited operators can use to reduce radiation exposure to patients.

   1. _____

   2. _____

   3. _____

   4. _____

2. A gonad shield must have a lead equivalency of at least:

   _____ .

3. The two radiology procedures with the greatest risk for occupational exposures are those involving:

   1. _____

   2. _____

4. Explain the differences between the long-term and short-term somatic effects of radiation.

   _____

   _____

   _____

   _____

   _____

5. The three principal methods used to protect limited operators from unnecessary radiation exposure are:

   1. _____

   2. _____

   3. _____

6. At what radiation dose would you see the first signs of a biologic effect? What would that effect be?

   _____

   _____

   _____

   _____

7. Name three reasons why the optically stimulated luminescence (OSL) personal dosimeter is the most commonly used dosimeter.

   1. _____

   2. _____

   3. _____

8. What should a limited operator do to minimize the need for repeat examinations?

_____

_____

_____

_____

_____

_____

_____

_____

9. What is meant by *low-dose technique?*

_____

_____

_____

_____

10. What is the limited operator's responsibility for ensuring that an embryo is not inadvertently exposed to x-rays?

_____

_____

_____

_____

_____

11. What is the primary method used to provide radiation safety for limited operators?

_____

_____

12. What is the lead equivalency of aprons and gloves worn by limited operators?

1. Aprons: _____

2. Gloves: _____

13. What does ALARA mean?

_____

14. Define *ionizing radiation*.

_____

_____

_____

15. Define *radiation protection*.

_____

_____

_____

16. Where should the radiation badge be worn?

_____

_____

17. Genetic effects and mutations are the results of radiation to which part of the body?

_____

18. The average person living in the United States is exposed to an annual dose of how much radiation?

_____

19. Describe the purpose of the control badge that comes with the personal dosimeters.

_____

CHALLENGE EXERCISE

This exercise does not have to be completed at the same time as the other exercises in this workbook chapter. The exercise is designed to assess retention of the essential information contained in the corresponding textbook chapter. It is recommended that you complete this exercise when you begin to study for the state limited licensure examination. This will help determine what you know and which information should be further reviewed.

1. The unit of radiation *exposure* is the:

_____.

2. The amount of x-rays absorbed by the irradiated tissue, or patient, is called the:

_____.

3. The absorbed dose in the body based on the type and energy of matter is called the:

_____.

4. X-ray photons have a radiation weighting factor of:

_____.

5. The measurement units of *exposure*, *absorbed dose*, and *equivalent dose* are:

Exposure: _____

Absorbed dose: _____

Equivalent dose: _____

6. Convert 0.10 Gy-$_a$ to mGy-$_a$.

_____

7. In our everyday work, the *equivalent dose* is used for:

_____.

8. Describe ESE.

_____.

9. The law of Bergonié–Tribondeau tells us what about radiation exposure?

_____.

10. Name the four characteristics of the law of Bergonié–Tribondeau.

1. _____

2. _____

3. _____

4. _____

11. Describe the radiation sensitivity difference between a younger patient's cells and an older patient's cells.

_____

12. Describe the radiation sensitivity difference between simple cells and highly complex cells.

_____

13. Name several cells in the body that would be very sensitive to radiation.

_____

14. Name several cells in the body that would *not* be very sensitive to radiation.

_____

15. Name four ways in which radiation effects in the body are classified.

    1. _____

    2. _____

    3. _____

    4. _____

16. Which radiation effect would be seen in about 3 months?

    _____

17. *Long-term* effects from radiation exposure are often referred to as:

    _____.

18. In diagnostic radiology, we are most concerned about which radiation effect?

    _____

19. When radiation damage affects the reproductive cells of the irradiated person, this effect is the:

    _____.

20. An observable *short-term* effect of radiation exposure is called:

    _____.

21. Describe the lethal dose (LD) 50/30.

    _____

22. What is the LD for human beings?

    _____

23. How much radiation does the skin have to receive for an erythema to develop?

    _____

24. Which effect of radiation exposure is not predictable?

    _____

25. Name at least four *long-term* somatic effects from radiation exposure.

    1. _____

    2. _____

    3. _____

    4. _____

26. The greatest percentage of *long-term* effects of radiation exposure will be seen in how many years?

_____

27. Which effect from radiation exposure will cause mutations in babies?

_____

28. Which body part should be protected with a lead shield to prevent mutations?

_____

29. Mutations caused by radiation exposure may be seen in a baby as:

   1. _____

   2. _____

   3. _____

30. How much radiation is the average person living in the United States exposed to?

_____

31. Describe the ALARA principle.

_____

32. The greatest cause of unnecessary radiation to patients that can be controlled by limited operators is:

_____

33. Name four ways in which patients can be protected from unnecessary radiation.

   1. _____

   2. _____

   3. _____

   4. _____

34. Gonad shields are used to reduce the likelihood of:

_____

35. The two categories of gonad shields are:

   1. _____

   2. _____

36. Gonad shields must be used when the primary x-ray beam is near the gonads. The dose will be significantly reduced with a shield when the radiation field is within:

_____.

37. The greatest risks of occupational exposure to radiation occur when the operator is working in which two areas of radiography?

    1. _____

    2. _____

38. The three principal methods used to protect limited operators from unnecessary radiation exposure are:

    1. _____

    2. _____

    3. _____

39. Lead aprons and gloves must have a quality control check every:

_____.

40. The lead-equivalency of aprons and gloves must be:

    Aprons: _____

    Gloves: _____

41. OSL personal dosimeters have what advantages?

    1. _____

    2. _____

    3. _____

    4. _____

42. What is the purpose of the control badge that comes with the department's personal dosimeters?

_____.

43. Where should personal dosimeters be worn?

_____.

44. The upper limit of occupational exposure, as determined by the National Council on Radiation Protection and Measurements (NCRP), is called the:

_____.

45. The lifetime risk of occupational exposure is referred to as the:

_____.

46. What is the maximum *effective dose* that an occupational worker can receive in 1 year?

_____

47. What is the formula for determining the *cumulative effective dose?*

_____

48. What is the *cumulative effective dose* for a 42-year-old occupational worker?

_____

49. NCRP studies confirm that a pregnant woman exposed to radiation in excess of _____ to the uterus is a cause for concern for the fetus.

50. The greatest risk to a fetus exists during which portion of pregnancy?

_____

51. The NCRP recommended monthly *equivalent dose* limit to the embryo or fetus for a pregnant worker is:

_____.

52. The NCRP recommended "9-month" *equivalent dose* limit to the embryo or fetus for a pregnant worker is:

_____.

53. When a pregnant worker wears a second personal dosimeter, where is it worn?

_____

12 Introduction to Anatomy, Positioning, and Pathology

EXERCISE 1

Answer the following questions by selecting the best choice.

1. The study of diseases that cause abnormal changes in the structure or function of body tissues and organs is called:
   A. anatomy.
   B. physiology.
   C. pathology.
   D. inflammation.

2. Which of the following is *not* an example of a tissue?
   A. Neuron
   B. Muscle
   C. Skin
   D. Stomach

3. Bone tissue that has a "honeycomb," or trabecular, structure is called:
   A. cartilage.
   B. marrow.
   C. cancellous tissue.
   D. cortex.

4. The elbow joint is an example of what type of joint?
   A. Synarthrodial joint
   B. Ball-and-socket joint
   C. Amphiarthrodial joint
   D. Diarthrodial joint

5. When a limb is moved toward the central part of the body, this motion is called:
   A. extension.
   B. aversion.
   C. adduction.
   D. abduction.

6. A position in which the patient is lying face up is called:
   A. supine.
   B. anatomic.
   C. prone.
   D. lateral decubitus.

7. When the patient is prone or facing the image receptor (IR), the projection is:
   A. anteroposterior (AP).
   B. posteroanterior (PA).
   C. lateral.
   D. oblique.

8. A disease that is relatively severe and that is characterized by a sudden onset and a short duration is described as:
   A. acute.
   B. chronic.
   C. exogenous.
   D. anomalous.

9. All of the following signs and symptoms may be typical of an inflammatory process *except:*
   A. pain.
   B. edema.
   C. heat at the site.
   D. ischemia.

10. All of the following conditions are classified as a neoplasm *except:*
    A. carcinoma.
    B. sarcoma.
    C. nosocomial disorder.
    D. lipoma.

Answer the following questions.

1. Name the three main parts of a cell.

    1. _____

    2. _____

    3. _____

2. Name three structures of the body that are composed of connective tissue.

    1. _____

    2. _____

    3. _____

3. What is the difference between a tissue and an organ?

    _____

    _____

4. Name two organs that are part of the respiratory system.

    1. _____

    2. _____

5. Describe the function of the skeletal system.

    _____

    _____

6. What is the hard, outer portion of most bones called? What is the inner, honeycomb portion called?

    _____

    _____

7. List the three classifications of joints and give an example of each.

    1. _____

    2. _____

    3. _____

8. Define the following terms used to describe joint motion.

abduct: _____

adduct: _____

extend: _____

flex: _____

pronate: _____

supinate: _____

9. Name the joint that is proximal to the hands and distal to the shoulders.

_____

10. What is the radiographic term for a body position in which the patient is lying on the left side?

_____

11. What is the name, and its abbreviation, for the projection in which the central ray enters the anterior surface and exits the posterior surface of the body?

_____

12. When the patient is lying on the left side and the central ray is vertical, what is the name of the projection?

_____

13. What phase of respiration does the patient hold for chest radiography? For abdominal radiography?

_____

14. Because the width of the clavicle is greater than its height, what is the correct IR orientation for an AP projection of the clavicle?

_____

15. List two endogenous conditions and two exogenous conditions.

Endogenous:

1. _____

2. _____

Exogenous:

1. _____

2. _____

16. List the four characteristics of inflammation.

1. _____

2. _____

3. _____

4. _____

17. Explain the differences between (1) acute and chronic conditions, and between (2) benign and malignant conditions.

1. _____

_____

2. _____

_____

18. What kinds of conditions are named with terms that end with *-itis* and *-oma?*

-itis: _____

-oma: _____

CHALLENGE EXERCISE

This exercise does not have to be completed at the same time as the other exercises in this workbook chapter. The exercise is designed to assess retention of the essential information contained in the corresponding textbook chapter. It is recommended that you complete this exercise when you begin to study for the state limited licensure examination. This will help determine what you know and which information should be further reviewed.

1. Define *anterior* as it relates to radiographic positioning. _____

_____

2. Define *posterior* as it relates to radiographic positioning. _____

_____

3. Define *cephalad* as it relates to radiographic positioning. _____

_____

4. Define *caudad* as it relates to radiographic positioning.

_____

5. Define *superior* as it relates to radiographic positioning. _____

_____

6. Define *inferior* as it relates to radiographic positioning. _____

_____

7. Define *internal* as it relates to radiographic positioning. _____

_____

8. Define *external* as it relates to radiographic positioning. _____

_____

9. Define *medial* as it relates to radiographic positioning. _____

_____

10. Define *lateral* as it relates to radiographic positioning. _____

_____

11. Define *proximal* as it relates to radiographic positioning. _____

_____

12. Define *distal* as it relates to radiographic positioning. _____

_____

13. Define *supine* as it relates to radiographic positioning. _____

_____

14. Define *prone* as it relates to radiographic positioning. _____

_____

15. Define *recumbent* as it relates to radiographic positioning. _____

_____

16. Define *upright* as it relates to radiographic positioning. _____

_____

17. Define *decubitus position* as it relates to radiographic positioning. _____

_____

18. Define *lateral position* as it relates to radiographic positioning. _____

_____

19. Define *oblique position* as it relates to radiographic positioning. _____

_____

13. A PA projection of the shoulder region in which the central ray is directed 30 degrees caudad is taken to demonstrate:
    A. fracture of the proximal humerus.
    B. the clavicle.
    C. the glenohumeral articulation.
    D. the acromioclavicular articulations.

14. To demonstrate a suspected fracture or dislocation in the shoulder region, the radiographic examination should consist of two projections: an AP taken with the coronal plane of the body parallel to the IR and a(n):
    A. AP projection in external rotation.
    B. AP projection in internal rotation.
    C. PA oblique projection (scapular Y).
    D. Grashey method projection.

15. The fat pad sign may be the only radiographic indication of:
    A. a scaphoid fracture.
    B. an elbow fracture.
    C. a glenohumeral dislocation.
    D. osteomyelitis.

16. The most common type of chronic degenerative joint disease that causes hypertrophy of the bone is:
    A. osteomyelitis.
    B. osteochondroma.
    C. osteoarthritis.
    D. osteoma.

EXERCISE 2

Label the following illustrations.

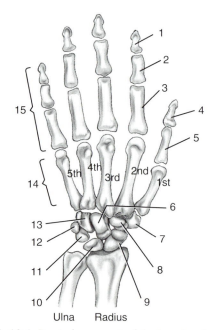

FIG. 13.1 Posterior aspect of the hand and wrist.

1. _____

2. _____

3. _____

4. _____

5. _____

6. _____

7. _____

8. _____

9. _____

10. _____

11. _____

12. _____

13. _____

14. _____

15. _____

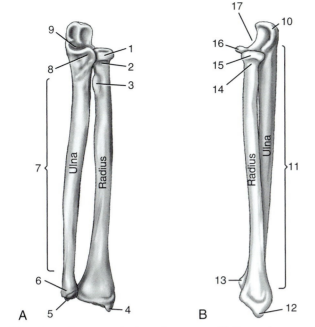

FIG. 13.2 Forearm. **A,** Anterior aspect. **B,** Lateral aspect.

1. _____

2. _____

3. _____

4. _____

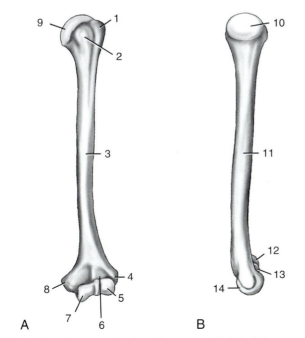

FIG. 13.3 Humerus. **A,** Anterior aspect. **B,** Medial aspect.

5. _____

6. _____

7. _____

8. _____

9. _____

10. _____

11. _____

12. _____

13. _____

14. _____

15. _____

16. _____

17. _____

1. _____

2. _____

3. _____

4. _____

5. _____

6. _____

7. _____

8. _____

9. _____

10. _____

11. _____

12. _____

13. _____

14. _____

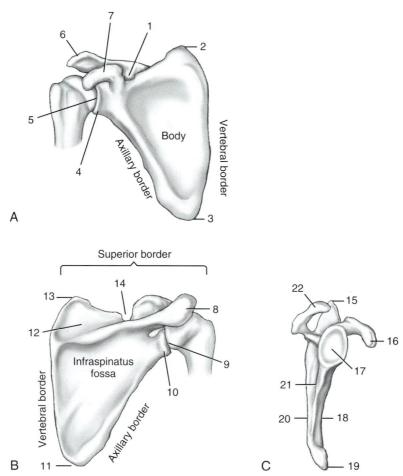

FIG. 13.4 Scapula. **A,** Anterior aspect. **B,** Posterior aspect. **C,** Lateral aspect.

1. _____

2. _____

3. _____

4. _____

5. _____

6. _____

7. _____

8. _____

9. _____

10. _____

11. _____

12. _____

13. _____

14. _____

15. _____

16. _____

17. _____

18. _____

19. _____

20. _____

21. _____

22. _____

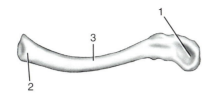

FIG. 13.5 Anterior aspect of the clavicle.

1. _____

2. _____

3. _____

FIG. 13.6 Palpable bony landmarks of the upper limb.

1. _____

2. _____

3. _____

4. _____

5. _____

6. _____

7. _____

8. _____

9. _____

10. _____

EXERCISE 3

Answer the following questions.

1. Name (1) the middle bone of the third digit, and (2) a carpal bone that articulates with the first metacarpal.

    1. _____

    2. _____

2. Is the ulna medial or lateral to the radius?

   _____

3. Name the articular processes of the distal humerus.

   _____

   _____

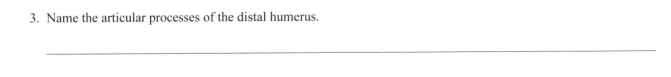

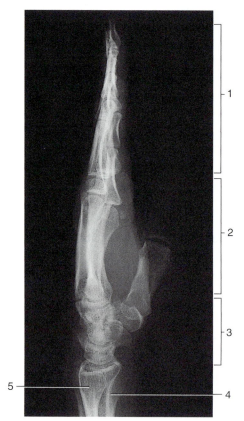

FIG. 13.8 Hand. Lateral projection.

1. _____
2. _____
3. _____
4. _____
5. _____

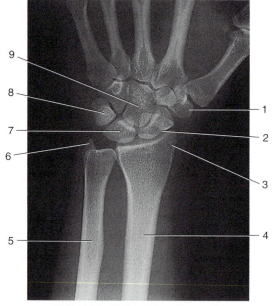

FIG. 13.9 Wrist. PA radiograph.

1. _____
2. _____
3. _____
4. _____
5. _____
6. _____
7. _____
8. _____
9. _____

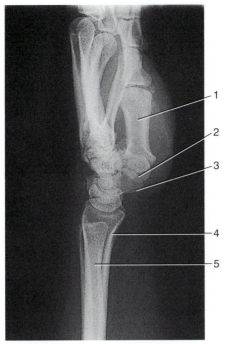

FIG. 13.10 Wrist. Lateral projection.

1. _____

2. _____

3. _____

4. _____

5. _____

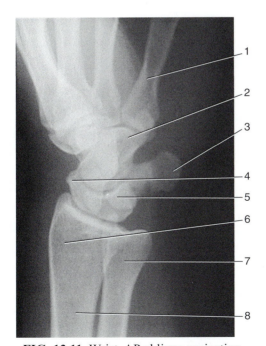

FIG. 13.11 Wrist. AP oblique projection.

1. _____

2. _____

3. _____

4. _____

5. _____

6. _____

7. _____

8. _____

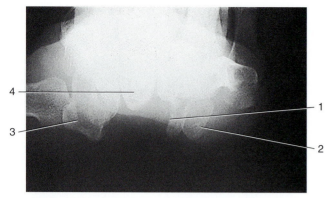

FIG. 13.12 Carpal canal. Tangential projection.

1. _____

2. _____

3. _____

4. _____

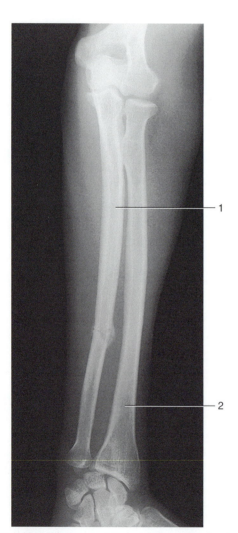

FIG. 13.13 Forearm. AP projection with fracture.

1. _____

2. _____

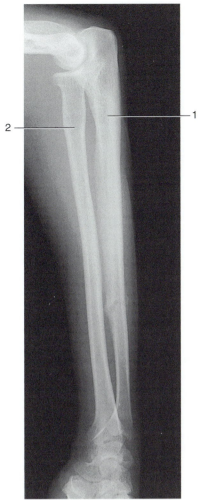

FIG. 13.14 Forearm. Lateral projection with fracture.

1. _____

2. _____

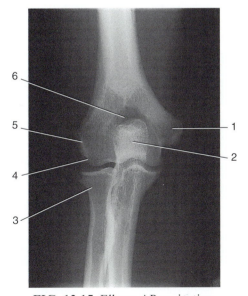

FIG. 13.15 Elbow. AP projection.

1. _____

2. _____

3. _____

4. _____

5. _____

6. _____

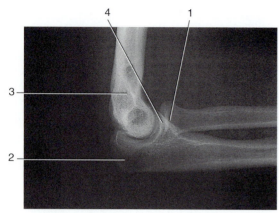

FIG. 13.16 Elbow. Lateral projection.

1. _____

2. _____

3. _____

4. _____

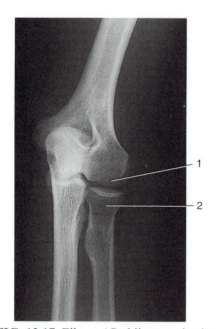

FIG. 13.17 Elbow. AP oblique projection.

1. _____

2. _____

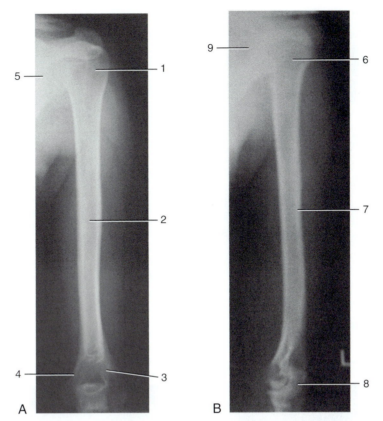

FIG. 13.18 Humerus. **A,** AP projection. **B,** Lateral projection.

1. _____

2. _____

3. _____

4. _____

5. _____

6. _____

7. _____

8. _____

9. _____

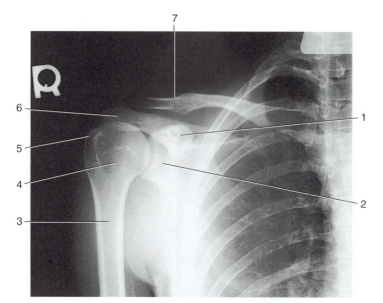

FIG. 13.19 Shoulder. AP projection, external arm rotation.

1. _____

2. _____

3. _____

4. _____

5. _____

6. _____

7. _____

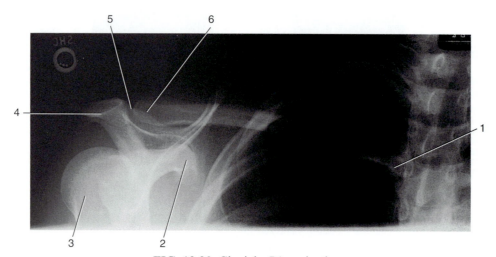

FIG. 13.20 Clavicle. PA projection.

1. _____

2. _____

3. _____

4. _____

5. _____

6. _____

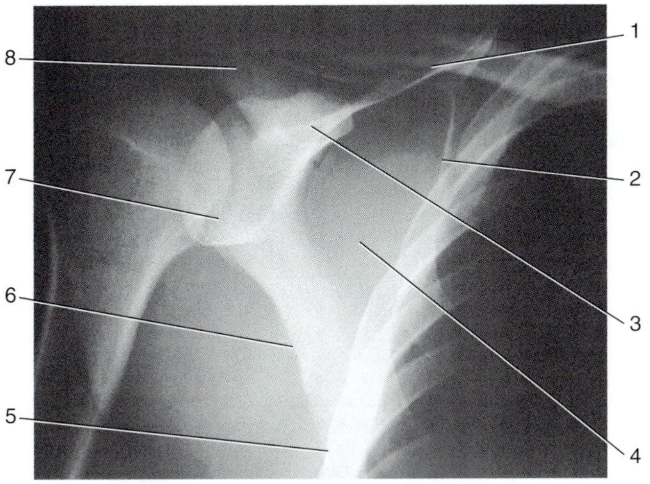

FIG. 13.21 Scapula. AP projection.

1. _____

2. _____

3. _____

4. _____

5. _____

6. _____

7. _____

8. _____

CHALLENGE EXERCISE

This exercise does not have to be completed at the same time as the other exercises in this workbook chapter. The exercise is designed to assess retention of the essential information contained in the corresponding textbook chapter. It is recommended that you complete this exercise when you begin to study for the state limited licensure examination. This will help determine what you know and which information should be further reviewed.

1. What is the minimum source–image receptor distance (SID) used for nearly all radiographic images of the upper limb?

   _____

2. Describe the positioning details for the PA projection of the hand. _____

   _____

3. What is the amount of lateral rotation needed to achieve a PA oblique projection of the hand?

   _____

   _____

4. Describe the positioning details for the PA oblique projection of the fourth (ring) finger.

   _____

   _____

5. Why is the PA projection *not* the routine projection for the thumb? _____

   _____

6. Describe the positioning details for the PA projection of the wrist. _____

   _____

7. Describe the positioning details for the lateral projection of the wrist. _____

_____

8. Describe the positioning details for the AP projection of the forearm. _____

_____

9. Describe the positioning details for the AP projection of the elbow. _____

_____

10. What is the degree of flexion needed for the lateral projection of the elbow? _____

_____

11. Describe the positioning details for the AP projection of the humerus. _____

_____

12. When performing an AP projection of the shoulder, what is the orientation of the coronal plane of the humeral epi-
    condyles to achieve external rotation of the humerus? _____

_____

13. When performing an AP projection of the shoulder, what is the orientation of the coronal plane of the humeral epi-
    condyles to achieve internal rotation of the humerus?

_____

_____

14. What are the amount and direction of central ray angulation for an AP axial projection of the clavicle?

_____

15. Why is it necessary to attach weights to the patient's wrists when performing radiography of the acromioclavicular
    joints?

_____

_____

14 Lower Limb and Pelvis

EXERCISE 1

Answer the following questions by selecting the best choice.

1. The bones of the midfoot consist of the:
   A. phalanges.
   B. tarsals.
   C. metatarsals.
   D. sesamoid bones.

2. Small, flat, oval bones in the region of the first metatarsophalangeal joint are called:
   A. phalanges.
   B. tarsals.
   C. metatarsals.
   D. sesamoid bones.

3. The sesamoid bone that is anterior to the distal femur and is commonly known as the *kneecap* is the:
   A. fibula.
   B. tibia.
   C. patella.
   D. fabella.

4. The ilium, ischium, and pubis join to form a synarthrodial joint at the:
   A. acetabulum.
   B. ilium.
   C. pubic symphysis.
   D. sacroiliac joint.

5. The palpable positioning landmark on the anterolateral aspect of the lateral pelvis above the hip is called the:
   A. anterior superior iliac spine.
   B. pubic symphysis.
   C. greater trochanter.
   D. ischial tuberosity.

6. When performing an anteroposterior (AP) axial projection of the foot, the central ray is directed:
   A. 10 degrees toward the toes.
   B. 10 degrees toward the heel.
   C. 15 degrees toward the heel.
   D. perpendicular to the image receptor (IR).

7. When the leg is extended, the ankle is dorsiflexed to form an angle of 90 degrees between the foot and leg, the leg is rotated medially approximately 15 to 20 degrees, and the central ray is perpendicular to the IR through the midpoint between the malleoli, the resulting image will demonstrate:

   A. an axial projection of the calcaneus.
   B. a medial oblique projection of the tarsals and metatarsals.
   C. the ankle mortise.
   D. the cuboid and the third cuneiform.

8. When the leg is extended in the supine position, the foot is maximally dorsiflexed, and the central ray is directed 40 degrees cephalad through the sole of the foot entering near the third metatarsal base, the resulting image will demonstrate:
   A. an axial projection of the calcaneus.
   B. a medial oblique projection of the tarsals and metatarsals.
   C. the cuboid and the third cuneiform.
   D. distal portions of the tibia and fibula.

9. Which of the following projections requires a central ray that is angled 5 to 7 degrees cephalad?
   A. An AP projection of the ankle
   B. A lateral projection of the knee
   C. An AP projection of the foot
   D. An axial projection of the calcaneus

10. When the patient is prone, the knee is flexed to form an angle of 75 to 80 degrees between the femur and the lower leg, and the central ray is directed approximately 15 to 20 degrees cephalad through the inferior margin of the patella, the resulting radiograph will demonstrate:
    A. a tangential projection of the patella.
    B. the patella in profile.
    C. the patellofemoral joint.
    D. all of the above.

11. When there is suspicion of a fracture of the patella, flexion of the knee joint for the lateral projection should be limited to:
    A. 5 to 7 degrees.
    B. 10 degrees.
    C. 20 to 30 degrees.
    D. 30 to 45 degrees.

12. When an AP projection of the proximal femur is performed, the IR should be placed so that the:
    A. superior margin is at the level of the greater trochanter.
    B. superior margin is at the level of the iliac crest.
    C. superior margin is at the level of the anterior superior iliac spine.
    D. center is aligned to the midfemur.

123

13. When an AP projection of the pelvis is performed and there is no suspicion of a recent fracture, the femurs are:
    A. rotated laterally 15 degrees.
    B. rotated medially 15 degrees.
    C. abducted maximally.
    D. maintained in a neutral AP position.

14. When a lateral projection is needed in cases of a known or suspected hip fracture, which projection(s) would be substituted for the frog-leg position?
    A. Axiolateral projection (Danelius–Miller method)
    B. Cross-table lateral projection
    C. Surgical lateral projection
    D. All of the above

15. A systemic disorder that increases the uric acid content of the blood and may cause a joint condition that commonly affects the feet (particularly the joints of the great toe) is called:
    A. osteoarthritis.
    B. gout.
    C. rheumatoid arthritis.
    D. osteoporosis.

16. _____ may cause degeneration of any of the joints of the lower limb but is most common in the knee and the hip.
    A. Osteoarthritis
    B. Osteomyelitis
    C. Osteogenic sarcoma
    D. Osteoporosis

EXERCISE 2

Answer the following questions.

1. How many phalanges are there in the great toe? The second toe?

   _____

   _____

2. Is the fibula medial or lateral to the tibia?

   _____

3. Name the bones that form the knee joint.

   _____

   _____

4. Name and point to three bony prominences on your own pelvis.

   1. _____

   2. _____

   3. _____

5. List two ways in which an examination of the foot differs from an examination of the ankle.

   1. _____

   _____

   2. _____

   _____

6. Describe the position of the leg for an AP oblique projection (mortise joint) of the ankle.

_____

_____

_____

7. Name two supplemental projections of the knee.

1. _____

2. _____

8. How does a routine hip examination differ from an examination for a possible hip fracture? Why?

_____

_____

_____

_____

_____

_____

_____

_____

9. List and describe four specific types of fractures of the lower limb and hip.

1. _____

_____

2. _____

_____

3. _____

_____

4. _____

_____

10. List three general types of nontraumatic pathology that may affect the bones of the lower limb or pelvis.

1. _____

2. _____

3. _____

EXERCISE 3

Label the following illustrations.

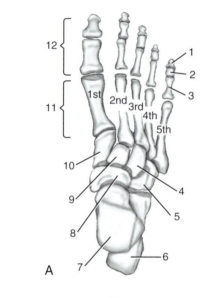

FIG. 14.1 Foot. **A,** Anterior (dorsal) aspect. **B,** Medial aspect.

1. _____

2. _____

3. _____

4. _____

5. _____

6. _____

7. _____

8. _____

9. _____

10. _____

11. _____

12. _____

13. _____

14. _____

15. _____

16. _____

17. _____

18. _____

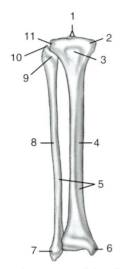

FIG. 14.2 Anterior aspect of the tibia and fibula.

1. _____

2. _____

3. _____

4. _____

5. _____

6. _____

7. _____

8. _____

9. _____

10. _____

11. _____

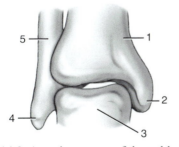

FIG. 14.3 Anterior aspect of the ankle joint.

1. _____

2. _____

3. _____

4. _____

5. _____

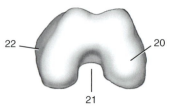

1. _____

2. _____

3. _____

4. _____

5. _____

6. _____

7. _____

8. _____

9. _____

10. _____

11. _____

12. _____

13. _____

14. _____

15. _____

16. _____

17. _____

18. _____

19. _____

20. _____

21. _____

22. _____

23. _____

24. _____

ANTERIOR ASPECT OF FEMUR   POSTERIOR ASPECT OF FEMUR

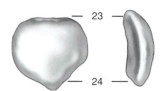

INFERIOR ASPECT OF FEMUR

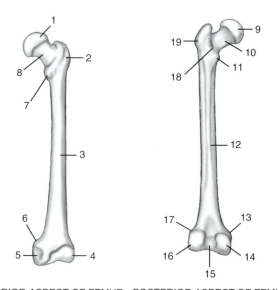

ANTERIOR ASPECT   LATERAL ASPECT
PATELLA

FIG. 14.4 Femur and patella.

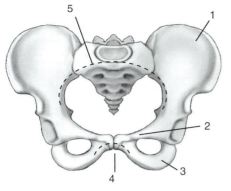

A   FEMALE PELVIS

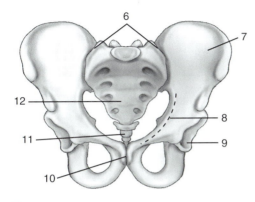

B   MALE PELVIS

FIG. 14.5 Pelvis. **A,** Female. **B,** Male.

1. _____

2. _____

3. _____

4. _____

5. _____

6. _____

7. _____

8. _____

9. _____

10. _____

11. _____

12. _____

EXERCISE 4

Label the following figures.

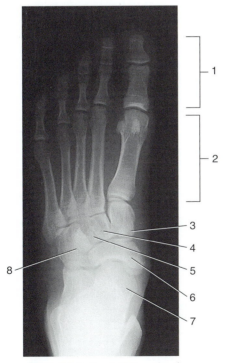

FIG. 14.6 Foot. AP projection.

1. _____

2. _____

3. _____

4. _____

5. _____

6. _____

7. _____

8. _____

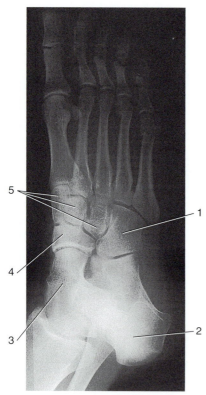

FIG. 14.7 Foot. AP oblique projection.

1. _____

2. _____

3. _____

4. _____

5. _____

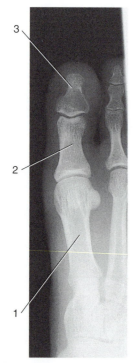

FIG. 14.8 Toes. AP projection.

1. _____

2. _____

3. _____

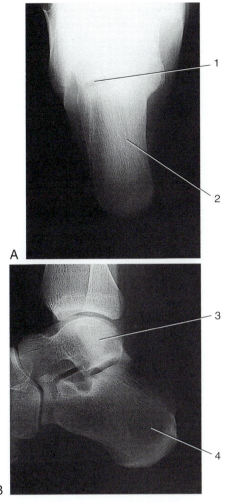

A

B

FIG. 14.9 Calcaneus. **A,** Axial projection. **B,** Lateral projection.

1. _____

2. _____

3. _____

4. _____

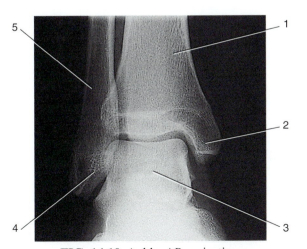

FIG. 14.10 Ankle. AP projection.

1. _____

2. _____

3. _____

4. _____

5. _____

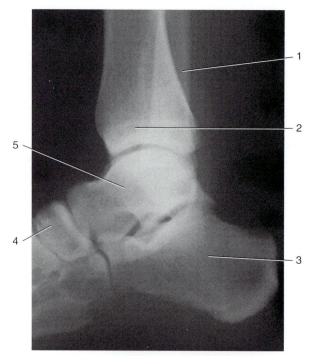

FIG. 14.11 Ankle. Lateral projection.

1. _____

2. _____

3. _____

4. _____

5. _____

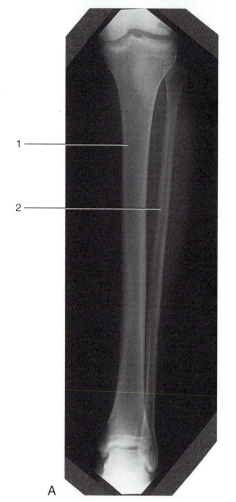

A

FIG. 14.12 Lower leg. **A,** AP projection.

1. _____

2. _____

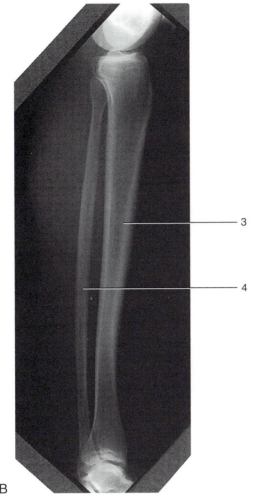

B

FIG. 14.12 Lower leg. **B,** Lateral projection.

3. _____

4. _____

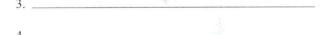

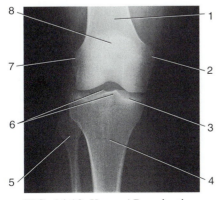

FIG. 14.13 Knee. AP projection.

1. _____

2. _____

3. _____

4. _____

5. _____

6. _____

7. _____

8. _____

CHALLENGE EXERCISE

This exercise does not have to be completed at the same time as the other exercises in this workbook chapter. The exercise is designed to assess retention of the essential information contained in the corresponding textbook chapter. It is recommended that you complete this exercise when you begin to study for the state limited licensure examination. This will help determine what you know and which information should be further reviewed.

1. What is the minimum source–image receptor distance (SID) used for nearly all radiography of the lower limb?

   _____

2. Describe the positioning details for the AP axial projection of the foot. _____

   _____

3. Describe the central ray placement for the AP axial projection of the foot. _____

   _____

4. What is the amount of medial rotation needed to achieve an AP oblique projection of the foot? _____

   _____

5. What are the amount and direction of central ray angulation for an axial (plantodorsal) projection of the calcaneus?

   _____

6. Describe the positioning details for the AP projection of the ankle. _____

   _____

7. Describe the central ray placement for the AP projection of the ankle. _____

   _____

8. Describe the positioning details for the lateral projection of the ankle. _____

   _____

9. Describe the central ray placement for the lateral projection of the ankle. _____

   _____

10. What are the amount and direction of leg rotation needed for an AP oblique projection of the ankle to demonstrate the distal tibiofibular joint?

    _____

11. What are the amount and direction of leg rotation needed for an AP oblique projection of the ankle to demonstrate the mortise joint?

    _____

12. Describe the positioning details for the AP projection of the knee. _____

_____

13. Describe the central ray placement for the AP projection of the knee. _____

_____

14. Describe the positioning details for the lateral projection of the knee. _____

_____

15. Describe the central ray placement for the lateral projection of the knee. _____

_____

16. Where is the superior margin of the IR or collimated field placed for an AP projection of the proximal femur?

_____

_____

17. Where is the inferior margin of the IR or collimated field placed for a lateral projection of the distal femur?

_____

_____

18. What are the amount and direction of leg rotation needed for an AP projection of the pelvis? _____

_____

19. What are the amount and direction of leg rotation needed for an AP projection of the hip? _____

_____

20. What is the amount of femur abduction needed for a lateral projection (frog-leg position) of the hip?

_____

15 Spine

EXERCISE 1

Answer the following questions by selecting the best choice.

1. The region of the spine that consists of five vertebrae and has a lordotic curve is the:
   A. cervical spine.
   B. thoracic spine.
   C. lumbar spine.
   D. sacrum.

2. The articular surfaces of the articular processes of the vertebrae are called:
   A. spinous processes.
   B. transverse processes.
   C. laminae.
   D. facets.

3. The blocklike anterior portion of a typical vertebra is called the:
   A. body.
   B. lamina.
   C. pedicle.
   D. articular process.

4. The number of vertebrae in the normal cervical spine is:
   A. 4.
   B. 5.
   C. 7.
   D. 12.

5. The axis is another name for:
   A. C1.
   B. C2.
   C. T1.
   D. L5.

6. The toothlike projection around which the atlas rotates is called the:
   A. axis.
   B. facet.
   C. articular process.
   D. dens or odontoid process.

7. When an anteroposterior (AP) projection of the cervical spine is performed, the central ray is directed:
   A. perpendicular to the image receptor (IR).
   B. 15 degrees caudad.
   C. 15 degrees cephalad.
   D. 25 degrees cephalad.

8. When the midsagittal plane of the body is parallel to the IR and the central ray is directed perpendicular to C4, the resulting image will be a(n):
   A. AP projection of the lower cervical spine.
   B. lateral projection of the cervical spine.
   C. anterior oblique projection of the cervical spine.
   D. AP projection of the upper cervical spine (open mouth).

9. A shallow breathing technique is used to advantage when taking a lateral projection of the:
   A. cervical spine.
   B. thoracic spine.
   C. lumbar spine.
   D. sacrum.

10. For which of the following projections is it most important to consider the anode heel effect when positioning the patient?
    A. AP projection of the lower cervical spine
    B. AP projection of the thoracic spine
    C. Lateral projection of the thoracic spine
    D. AP projection of the lumbar spine

11. A supine position with the central ray directed 10 degrees caudad 1 inch inferior to the anterior superior iliac spine is used to demonstrate an:
    A. AP axial projection of the lumbosacral joint.
    B. AP axial projection of the sacrum.
    C. AP axial projection of the coccyx.
    D. AP projection of the pelvis.

12. Spine radiography may be performed with the patient:
    A. upright.
    B. supine.
    C. prone.
    D. all of the above.

13. Patient breathing instructions for all projections of the lumbar spine should include:
    A. suspend breathing on inspiration.
    B. suspend breathing on expiration.
    C. breathe shallowly.
    D. all of the above.

14. The central ray for a lateral projection of the lumbar spine when using a 35- × 43-cm IR is:
    A. perpendicular to the IR through L4.
    B. perpendicular to the IR through L3.
    C. in the midaxillary line.
    D. both A and C.

15. The projection commonly called the *swimmer's technique* will demonstrate which region of the spine?
    A. Cervical region
    B. Cervicothoracic region
    C. Thoracic region
    D. Lumbar region

16. The positioning steps for the AP projection of the upper cervical spine open-mouth technique include which of the following?
    A. Align the midsagittal plane perpendicular to the IR.
    B. Align the occlusal plane and base of the skull parallel to the horizontal plane.
    C. Use close collimation.
    D. All of the above.

17. Which palpable landmark would be used when positioning for an AP projection of the lumbar spine?
    A. Iliac crest
    B. Jugular notch
    C. Xiphoid process
    D. Lower costal margin

18. When the posterior portions of the neural arch fail to close during early embryonic development, the condition is known as:
    A. spina bifida.
    B. meningomyelocele.
    C. herniated nucleus pulposus.
    D. stenosis.

19. Which region of the spine is the most common site of pathologic compression fractures of vertebral bodies due to osteoporosis?
    A. Cervical region
    B. Thoracic region
    C. Lumbar region
    D. Sacral region

20. Which of the following conditions is demonstrated by magnetic resonance imaging or computed tomography but is not normally seen on routine radiography?
    A. Compression fracture
    B. Spondylosis
    C. Spina bifida
    D. Disk herniation

EXERCISE 2

Answer the following questions.

1. List the sections of the spine and state the number of vertebrae or vertebral segments in each.

_____

_____

_____

_____

_____

2. Which spinal segments have a kyphotic curve? Which have a lordotic curve?

_____

_____

_____

_____

3. How do the atlas and axis differ from the other cervical vertebrae?

_____

_____

_____

4. On your own body, indicate the locations of the mental point, mastoid process, and angle of the mandible; laryngeal (thyroid cartilage) prominence; and jugular (sternal) notch.

_____

_____

_____

_____

5. An AP projection of the upper cervical spine is unsatisfactory because the patient's upper teeth are superimposed over the atlas and the dens. How should you adjust the position for a satisfactory radiograph?

_____

_____

_____

6. Name and describe positions that will demonstrate each of the following structures: the left cervical intervertebral foramina, the cervical zygapophyseal joints, the lumbar intervertebral foramina, the left lumbar zygapophyseal joints, and the sacroiliac joints.

_____

_____

_____

_____

_____

_____

7. An order for radiographic examination of the cervical spine includes a request for lateral flexion and extension positions. The patient was in a car accident this morning. What precautions are needed? Why?

_____

_____

_____

_____

_____

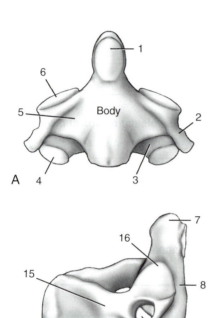

A

B

FIG. 15.3 Atlas. **A,** Anterior aspect. **B,** Lateral aspect.

1. _____
2. _____
3. _____
4. _____
5. _____
6. _____
7. _____
8. _____
9. _____
10. _____
11. _____
12. _____
13. _____
14. _____
15. _____
16. _____

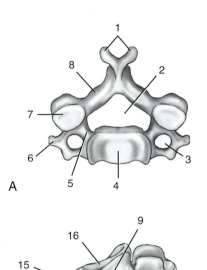

A

B

FIG. 15.4 Typical cervical vertebra. **A,** Superior aspect. **B,** Lateral aspect.

1. _____
2. _____
3. _____
4. _____
5. _____
6. _____
7. _____
8. _____
9. _____
10. _____
11. _____
12. _____
13. _____
14. _____
15. _____
16. _____

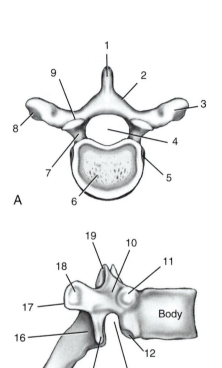

A

B

FIG. 15.5 Thoracic vertebra. **A,** Superior aspect. **B,** Lateral aspect.

Body

1. _____

2. _____

3. _____

4. _____

5. _____

6. _____

7. _____

8. _____

9. _____

10. _____

11. _____

12. _____

13. _____

14. _____

15. _____

16. _____

17. _____

18. _____

19. _____

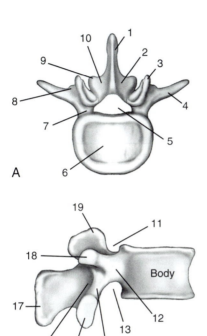

A

B

FIG. 15.6 Lumbar vertebra. **A,** Anterior aspect. **B,** Lateral aspect.

1. _____
2. _____
3. _____
4. _____
5. _____
6. _____
7. _____
8. _____
9. _____
10. _____
11. _____
12. _____
13. _____
14. _____
15. _____
16. _____
17. _____
18. _____
19. _____

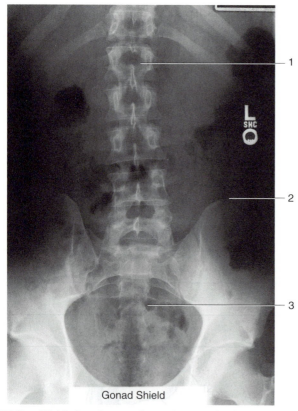

FIG. 15.10 Lumbar spine. AP projection, patient recumbent with knees flexed.

1. _____

2. _____

3. _____

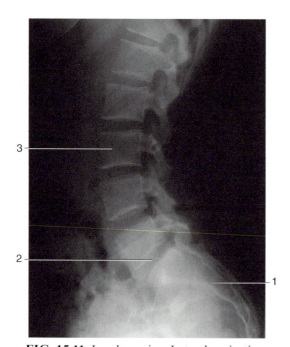

FIG. 15.11 Lumbar spine. Lateral projection.

1. _____

2. _____

3. _____

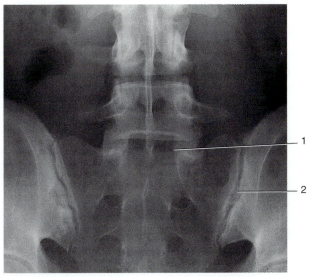

FIG. 15.12 Lumbosacral junction and sacroiliac joints. AP axial projection.

1. _____

2. _____

CHALLENGE EXERCISE

This exercise does not have to be completed at the same time as the other exercises in this workbook chapter. The exercise is designed to assess retention of the essential information contained in the corresponding textbook chapter. It is recommended that you complete this exercise when you begin to study for the state limited licensure examination. This will help determine what you know and which information should be further reviewed.

1. Describe the positioning details for the AP axial projection of the lower cervical spine.

   _____

   _____

2. Describe the central ray angle and placement for the AP axial projection of the lower cervical spine.

   _____

3. Describe the positioning details for the AP projection of the upper cervical spine.

   _____

   _____

4. Describe the central ray angle and placement for the AP projection of the upper cervical spine.

   _____

5. Describe the positioning details for the lateral projection of the cervical spine.

   _____

   _____

6. Describe the central ray angle and placement for the lateral projection of the cervical spine.

_____

7. What is the source–image receptor distance (SID) range used for the lateral projection of the cervical spine?

_____

8. Describe the positioning details for the AP axial oblique projection of the cervical spine.

_____

_____

9. Describe the central ray angle and placement for the AP axial oblique projection of the cervical spine.

_____

10. What is the common name for the lateral projection of the cervicothoracic region? Hint: You do it in the water.

_____

11. Describe how the "breathing technique" is performed for the lateral projection of the thoracic spine.

_____

_____

12. Describe the positioning details for the AP projection of the lumbar spine.

_____

_____

13. Describe the central ray angle and placement for the AP projection of the lumbar spine.

_____

14. Describe the positioning details for the lateral projection of the lumbar spine.

_____

_____

15. Describe the central ray angle and placement for the lateral projection of the lumbar spine.

_____

16. Describe the positioning details for the AP oblique projection of the lumbar spine.

_____

_____

17. Describe the central ray angle and placement for the AP oblique projection of the lumbar spine.

_____

18. What is the purpose of the lateral projection of the L5 to S1 lumbosacral junction?

_____

_____

19. Describe the positioning details for the AP oblique projection of the sacroiliac joint.

_____

_____

20. Describe the central ray angle and placement for the AP oblique projection of the sacroiliac joint.

_____

21. Describe the positioning details for the AP axial projection of the sacrum.

_____

_____

22. Describe the central ray angle and placement for the AP axial projection of the sacrum.

_____

23. Describe the central ray angle and placement for the AP axial projection of the coccyx.

_____

24. Describe the positioning details for the lateral projection of the sacrum.

_____

_____

25. Describe the central ray angle and placement for the lateral projection of the sacrum.

_____

16 Bony Thorax, Chest, and Abdomen

EXERCISE 1

Answer the following questions by selecting the best choice.

1. Which of the following terms does *not* refer to a portion of the sternum?
   A. Body
   B. Manubrium
   C. Mediastinum
   D. Xiphoid process

2. The lower five pairs of ribs are called:
   A. true ribs.
   B. false ribs.
   C. floating ribs.
   D. cervical ribs.

3. All of the following organs are found within the mediastinum *except* the:
   A. heart.
   B. lungs.
   C. trachea.
   D. ascending aorta.

4. The inferior lateral "corners" of the lungs are called the:
   A. hila.
   B. inferior lobes.
   C. cardiophrenic angles.
   D. costophrenic angles.

5. When the abdomen is divided into nine regions, the lower middle portion is called the:
   A. hypochondriac region.
   B. iliac region.
   C. hypogastric region.
   D. umbilical region.

6. The first and proximal portion of the small bowel is called the:
   A. duodenum.
   B. pylorus.
   C. jejunum.
   D. ileum.

7. The function(s) of the large intestine include:
   A. reclamation of water from intestinal contents.
   B. elimination of solid waste.
   C. production of bile.
   D. A and B.

8. Routine projections for the right fourth posterior rib, when the injury is posterior, are:
   A. posteroanterior (PA) and left anterior oblique (LAO).
   B. PA and right anterior oblique (RAO).
   C. anteroposterior (AP) and right posterior oblique (RPO).
   D. AP and left posterior oblique (LPO).

9. Routine projections for the left tenth anterior rib, when the injury is anterior, are:
   A. PA and LAO.
   B. PA and RAO.
   C. AP and RPO.
   D. AP and LPO.

10. When an AP projection of the abdomen is performed, the correct source–image receptor distance (SID) is:
    A. 40 inches.
    B. 48 inches.
    C. 60 inches.
    D. 72 inches.

11. Examination of the chest differs from examination of the ribs in that:
    A. a 72-inch SID is used.
    B. a higher peak kilovoltage (kVp) is used.
    C. exposure is made on expiration.
    D. both A and B.

12. An upright AP projection of the abdomen is useful for the visualization of:
    A. air–fluid levels in the intestines.
    B. liver size.
    C. kidney stones.
    D. diverticulosis.

13. When a PA projection of the chest is performed, the correct SID is:
    A. 40 inches.
    B. 48 inches.
    C. 60 inches.
    D. 72 inches.

14. Lateral projections of the chest are taken with the left side against the image receptor (IR) because:
    A. magnification of the cardiac silhouette is minimized with the left side nearer the IR.
    B. it is conventional to have a routine standard, and the left has been established as the standard.
    C. lung pathology is more common on the left side.
    D. the right hilum provides high-contrast details that may be confusing.

15. Which of the following techniques is desirable for chest radiography?
    A. High kVp, high milliamperes (mA), and short exposure time
    B. Low kVp and 72 inches SID
    C. Low kVp, high milliampere-seconds (mAs)
    D. High kVp, 72 inches SID, and low mA

16. Breathing instructions for the AP projection of the abdomen should include:
    A. suspend breathing on the first deep inspiration.
    B. suspend breathing on the second deep inspiration.
    C. suspend breathing on the first deep expiration.
    D. suspend breathing on the second deep expiration.

17. To demonstrate air–fluid levels in radiography, use:
    A. the decubitus position.
    B. the upright position.
    C. a horizontal x-ray beam.
    D. all of the above.

18. Breathing instructions for a PA projection of the chest should include:
    A. suspend breathing on the first deep inspiration.
    B. suspend breathing on the second deep inspiration.
    C. suspend breathing on the first deep expiration.
    D. suspend breathing on the second deep expiration.

19. Which of the following conditions is an inflammatory occupational lung disease caused by inhaling irritating dust?
    A. Tuberculosis
    B. Pneumoconiosis
    C. *Pneumocystis carinii* pneumonia
    D. Pneumothorax

20. All of the following abdominal features can be seen on noncontrast media studies of the abdomen, *except:*
    A. the outer contours of the kidneys.
    B. gas in the colon.
    C. the psoas muscle.
    D. the pancreas.

EXERCISE 2

Answer the following questions.

1. Name the parts of the sternum and point to each on your own body.

    _____

    _____

    _____

    _____

2. Make a simple drawing of a lung and indicate the apex, hilum, costophrenic angle, and cardiophrenic angle.

3. Name four structures located within the mediastinum and state the body system to which each belongs.

    1. _____

    2. _____

    3. _____

    4. _____

4. Name two organs found in each quadrant of the abdomen.

   Right upper quadrant: _____

   Left upper quadrant: _____

   Right lower quadrant: _____

   Left lower quadrant: _____

5. Name the projections that constitute a routine examination of the left upper anterior ribs and the right lower posterior ribs.

   _____

   _____

   _____

6. Should ribs below the diaphragm be exposed on inspiration or expiration?

   _____

7. List as many differences as you can between rib radiography and chest radiography.

   _____

   _____

   _____

   _____

   _____

   _____

8. If a patient with acute abdominal pain cannot stand for an upright AP abdominal projection, what projection should be substituted? Why is this important?

   _____

   _____

   _____

   _____

9. List three conditions that involve inflammation of the lungs.

   1. _____

   2. _____

   3. _____

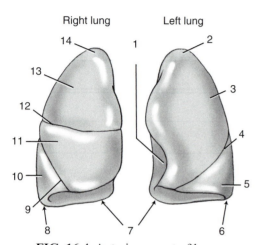

Right lung   Left lung

FIG. 16.4 Anterior aspect of lungs.

1. _____

2. _____

3. _____

4. _____

5. _____

6. _____

7. _____

8. _____

9. _____

10. _____

11. _____

12. _____

13. _____

14. _____

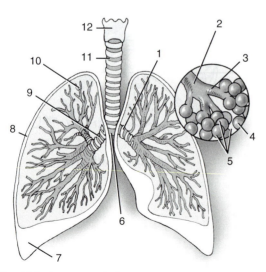

FIG. 16.5 Organs of the respiratory system in the thoracic cavity.

1. _____

2. _____

3. _____

4. _____

5. _____

6. _____

7. _____

8. _____

9. _____

10. _____

11. _____

12. _____

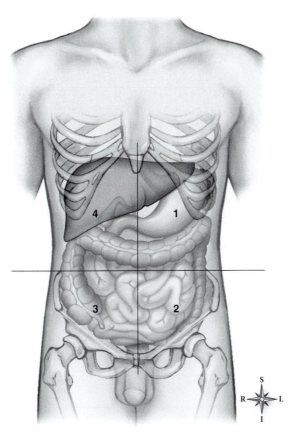

FIG. 16.6 Abdominopelvic cavity divided into quadrants.

1. _____

2. _____

3. _____

4. _____

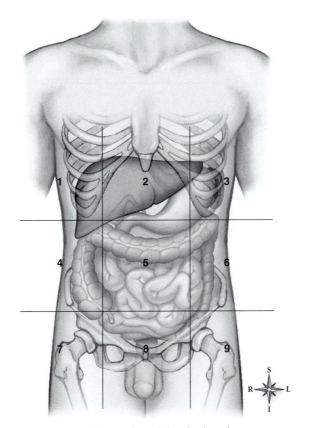

FIG. 16.7 Nine abdominal regions.

1. _____

2. _____

3. _____

4. _____

5. _____

6. _____

7. _____

8. _____

9. _____

161

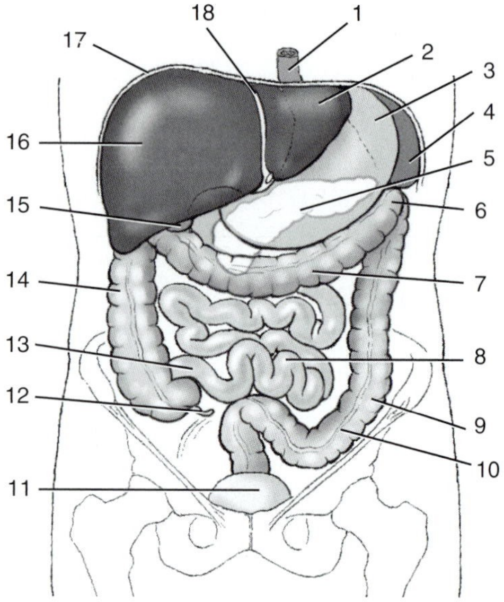

FIG. 16.8 Abdominal organs of the digestive system.

1. _____

2. _____

3. _____

4. _____

5. _____

6. _____

7. _____

8. _____

9. _____

10. _____

11. _____

12. _____

13. _____

14. _____

15. _____

16. _____

17. _____

18. _____

Label the following figures.

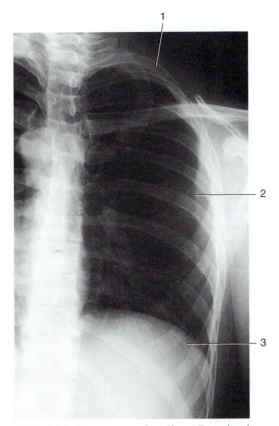

FIG. 16.9 Upper posterior ribs. AP projection.

1. _____

2. _____

3. _____

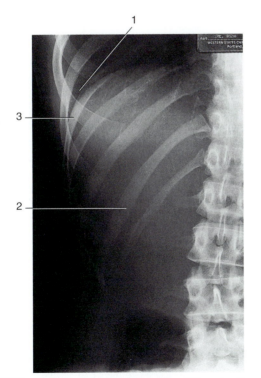

FIG. 16.10 Lower posterior ribs. AP projection.

1. _____

2. _____

3. _____

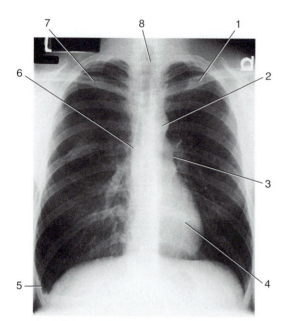

FIG. 16.11 Chest. PA projection.

1. _____

2. _____

3. _____

4. _____

5. _____

6. _____

7. _____

8. _____

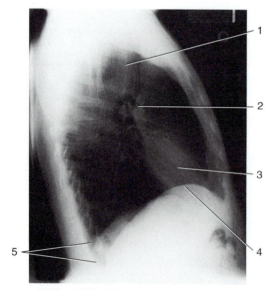

FIG. 16.12 Chest. Lateral projection.

1. _____

2. _____

3. _____

4. _____

5. _____

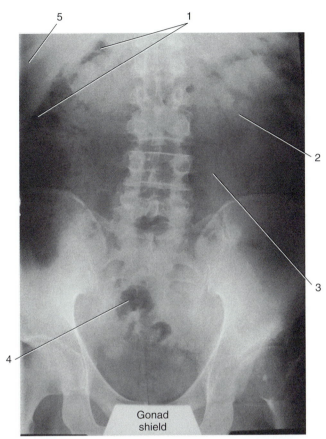

FIG. 16.13 Abdomen. AP projection, patient recumbent.

1. _____

2. _____

3. _____

4. _____

5. _____

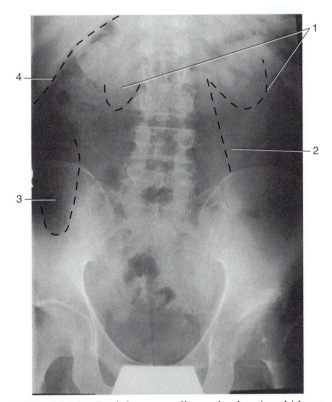

FIG. 16.14 AP abdomen radiograph showing kidney shadows, liver margin, and psoas muscles.

1. _____

2. _____

3. _____

4. _____

This exercise does not have to be completed at the same time as the other exercises in this workbook chapter. The exercise is designed to assess retention of the essential information contained in the corresponding textbook chapter. It is recommended that you complete this exercise when you begin to study for the state limited licensure examination. This will help determine what you know and which information should be further reviewed.

1. Describe the movement of the diaphragm during inspiration.

   _____

2. Describe the movement of the diaphragm during expiration.

   _____

3. What is the recommended SID for routine radiography of the chest?

   _____

4. Describe the positioning details for the PA projection of the chest.

   _____

   _____

5. Describe the central ray placement for the PA projection of the chest.

   _____

6. Describe the patient breathing instructions for the PA projection of the chest.

   _____

7. Describe the positioning details for the lateral projection of the chest.

   _____

   _____

8. Describe the central ray placement for the lateral projection of the chest.

   _____

9. Describe the positioning details for the AP projection (lateral decubitus position) of the chest.

   _____

   _____

10. Describe the positioning details for the AP oblique projection of the upper ribs.

    _____

    _____

11. Describe the patient breathing instructions for the AP oblique projection of the upper ribs.

_____

12. Describe the positioning details for the AP projection of the lower posterior ribs.

_____

_____

13. Describe the patient breathing instructions for the AP projection of the lower posterior ribs.

_____

14. Describe the positioning details for the AP projection of the abdomen.

_____

_____

15. Describe the patient breathing instructions for the AP projection of the abdomen.

_____

Answer the following questions.

1. Name the bones that make up the cranium.

   _____

   _____

   _____

2. Which cranial bones contain the auditory canals?

   _____

   _____

3. List the bones that make up the orbit.

   _____

   _____

   _____

4. List the bones that contain the paranasal sinuses.

   _____

   _____

   _____

5. Name a projection that demonstrates the cranial base.

   _____

   _____

   _____

6. Compare the procedure for an AP axial (Towne method) projection with the procedure for demonstrating the same structures with the patient prone.

   _____

   _____

   _____

   _____

   _____

   _____

7. Name two projections that demonstrate the maxillary sinuses.

   1. _____

   2. _____

8. How does the procedure for a lateral projection of the nasal bones differ from that for a lateral projection of the facial bones?

   _____

   _____

   _____

   _____

   _____

9. Describe the patient or part position for a parietoacanthial (Waters method) projection of the facial bones and sinuses.

   _____

   _____

   _____

   _____

10. If the petrous ridge is projected over the floor of the maxillary sinuses on the parietoacanthial (Waters method) projection, how should the position be modified to clearly demonstrate this area?

    _____

    _____

11. List three types of facial fractures and state the projection(s) most likely to provide a clear demonstration of each.

    1. _____

    2. _____

    3. _____

12. Name three types of pathologic conditions that may be diagnosed by radiography of the cranium.

    1. _____

    2. _____

    3. _____

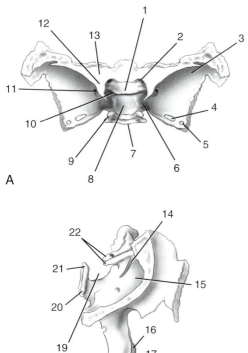

A

B

FIG. 17.2 Sphenoid bone. **A,** Superior aspect. **B,** Lateral aspect.

1. _____
2. _____
3. _____
4. _____
5. _____
6. _____
7. _____
8. _____
9. _____
10. _____
11. _____
12. _____
13. _____
14. _____
15. _____
16. _____
17. _____
18. _____
19. _____
20. _____
21. _____
22. _____

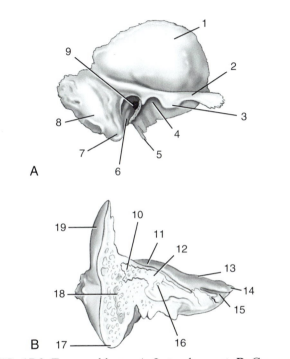

1. _____

2. _____

3. _____

4. _____

5. _____

6. _____

7. _____

8. _____

9. _____

10. _____

11. _____

12. _____

13. _____

14. _____

15. _____

16. _____

17. _____

18. _____

19. _____

FIG. 17.3 Temporal bone. **A,** Lateral aspect. **B,** Coronal section through mastoid and petrous portions.

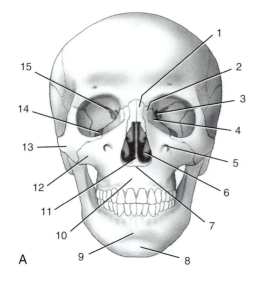

A

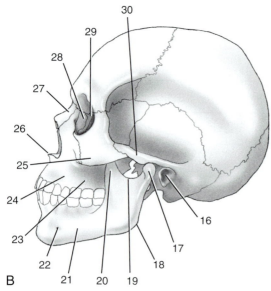

B

FIG. 17.4 Facial bones. **A,** Anterior aspect. **B,** Lateral aspect.

6. _____

7. _____

8. _____

9. _____

10. _____

11. _____

12. _____

13. _____

14. _____

15. _____

16. _____

17. _____

18. _____

19. _____

20. _____

21. _____

22. _____

23. _____

24. _____

25. _____

26. _____

27. _____

28. _____

29. _____

30. _____

1. _____

2. _____

3. _____

4. _____

5. _____

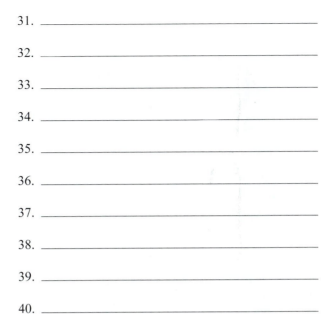

C

FIG. 17.4, cont'd Facial bones. **C,** Interior of facial bones, lateral aspect.

31. _____
32. _____
33. _____
34. _____
35. _____
36. _____
37. _____
38. _____
39. _____
40. _____

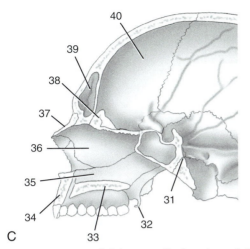

A

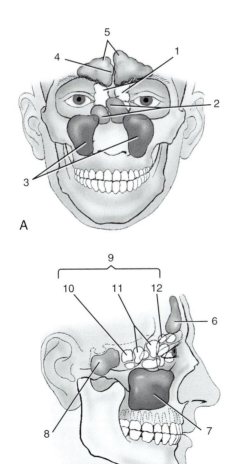

B

FIG. 17.5 Paranasal sinuses. **A,** Anterior aspect. **B,** Lateral aspect.

1. _____
2. _____
3. _____
4. _____
5. _____
6. _____
7. _____
8. _____
9. _____
10. _____
11. _____
12. _____

177

Label the following figures.

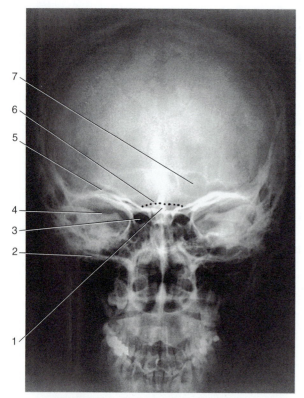

FIG. 17.6 Cranium. PA projection.

1. _____

2. _____

3. _____

4. _____

5. _____

6. _____

7. _____

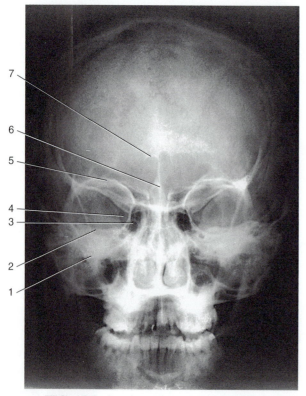

FIG. 17.7 Cranium. PA axial projection.

1. _____

2. _____

3. _____

4. _____

5. _____

6. _____

7. _____

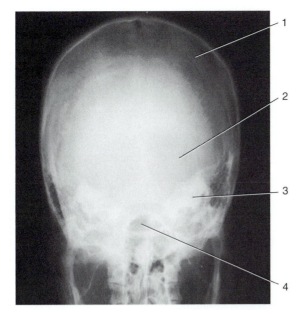

FIG. 17.8 Cranium. AP axial projection (Towne method).

1. _____

2. _____

3. _____

4. _____

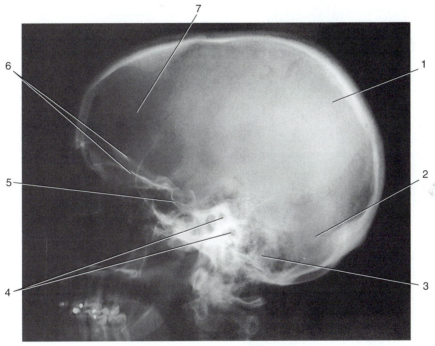

FIG. 17.9 Cranium. Lateral projection.

1. _____

2. _____

3. _____

4. _____

5. _____

6. _____

7. _____

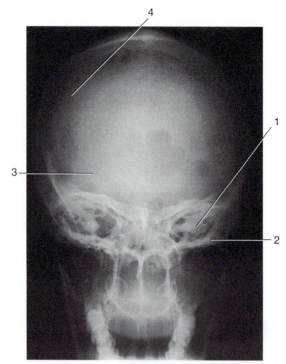

FIG. 17.10 Cranium. AP projection.

1. _____

2. _____

3. _____

4. _____

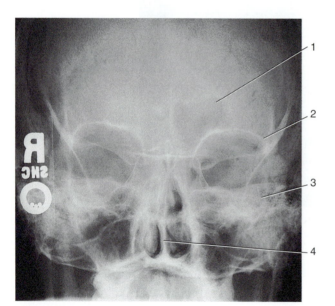

FIG. 17.11 Facial bones. PA axial projection (Caldwell method).

1. _____

2. _____

3. _____

4. _____

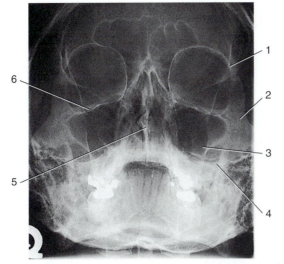

FIG. 17.12 Facial bones. Parietoacanthial projection (Waters method).

1. _____
2. _____
3. _____
4. _____
5. _____
6. _____

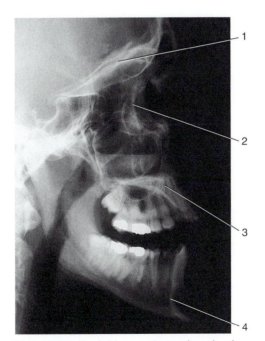

FIG. 17.13 Facial bones. Lateral projection.

1. _____
2. _____
3. _____
4. _____

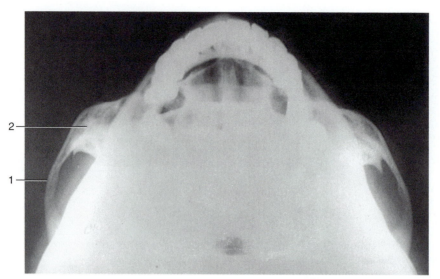

FIG. 17.14 Zygomatic arches. Verticosubmental projection.

1. _____

2. _____

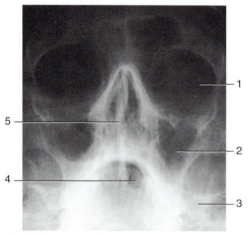

FIG. 17.15 Paranasal sinuses. Parietoacanthial projection (Waters method).

1. _____

2. _____

3. _____

4. _____

5. _____

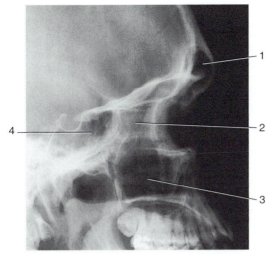

FIG. 17.16 Paranasal sinuses. Lateral projection.

1. _____
2. _____
3. _____
4. _____

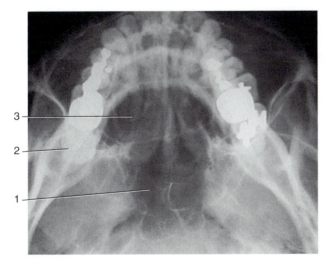

FIG. 17.17 Paranasal sinuses. Submentovertical projection.

1. _____
2. _____
3. _____

This exercise does not have to be completed at the same time as the other exercises in this workbook chapter. The exercise is designed to assess retention of the essential information contained in the corresponding textbook chapter. It is recommended that you complete this exercise when you begin to study for the state limited licensure examination. This will help determine what you know and which information should be further reviewed.

1. Describe the skull positioning landmark called the *glabella.*

   _____

2. Describe the skull positioning landmark called the *nasion.*

   _____

3. Describe the skull positioning landmark called the *acanthion.*

   _____

4. Describe the skull positioning landmark called the *mental point.*

   _____

5. Describe the skull positioning landmark called the *gonion.*

   _____

6. Describe the positioning details for the PA axial projection of the skull.

   _____

   _____

7. Describe the central ray placement for the PA axial projection of the skull.

   _____

8. Describe the positioning details for the AP axial projection of the skull.

   _____

   _____

9. Describe the central ray placement for the AP axial projection of the skull.

   _____

10. What positioning and central ray adjustments are needed for the AP axial projection of the skull if the patient is unable to flex the neck sufficiently to get the orbitomeatal line perpendicular to the IR?

   _____

   _____

11. Describe the positioning details for the lateral projection of the skull.

_____

_____

12. Describe the central ray placement for the lateral projection of the skull.

_____

13. Describe the positioning details for the parietoacanthial projection of the facial bones and sinuses.

_____

_____

14. Describe the central ray placement for the parietoacanthial projection of the facial bones and sinuses.

_____

15. Describe the central ray placement for the lateral projection of the facial bones.

_____

16. Why do all sinus radiographs need to be performed upright?

_____

17. Describe the positioning details for the PA axial projection of the sinuses.

_____

_____

18. Describe the central ray angle and placement for the AP axial projection of the mandible.

_____

19. Describe the positioning details for the PA axial projection of the mandible.

_____

_____

20. Describe the positioning details for the axiolateral projection of the mandible.

_____

_____

18 Radiography of Pediatric and Geriatric Patients

EXERCISE 1

Answer the following questions.

1. The term that refers to the care of older adults is _____.

2. The term that refers to the care of infants and children is _____.

3. List three things you might do to calm an infant.

    1. _____

    2. _____

    3. _____

4. (True/False) More information is communicated nonverbally than with words.

5. When a toddler is refusing to cooperate, what are two things you can do that might change the child's attitude?

    1. _____

    2. _____

6. Explain what is meant by a "valid choice."

    _____

    _____

7. (True/False) When a child is to have a radiographic examination, a parent should never be allowed in the x-ray room.

8. (True/False) Mechanical immobilization is preferable to having someone hold a child during an x-ray exposure.

9. (True/False) When a child must be held during an x-ray exposure, x-ray personnel should hold the child.

10. The principal objective when immobilizing an infant or child for radiography is _____

    _____.

11. Bilateral studies of the _____ and the _____ are seldom required for adults but are usually performed for children.

12. List three ways in which the anatomy of children differs from that of adults.

    1. _____

    2. _____

    3. _____

5. A currently used term for physical child abuse or battered child syndrome is _____

   _____

6. Lack of bone density in the aged is referred to as *demineralization* or

   _____

7. A characteristic of Parkinson disease that creates problems during radiography is

   _____

8. What age group is most commonly affected by the condition known as *organic brain syndrome?*

   _____

9. Black eyes, bulging fontanels, or unexplained unconsciousness in an infant should raise suspicion of

   _____

10. Decubitus ulcers most commonly occur in the elderly and the bedridden as a result of

    _____

    _____

19 Image Evaluation

EXERCISE 1

Answer the following questions by selecting the best choice.

1. Image evaluation is the process that determines whether an image:
   1. is correctly identified and marked.
   2. contains sufficient diagnostic quality.
   3. meets the minimum requirements of the imaging order.
   A. 1 and 2
   B. 1 and 3
   C. 2 and 3
   D. 1, 2, and 3

2. Which of the following conditions should be observed when viewing radiographs?
   1. View each with a bright light.
   2. Maintain a clean monitor screen.
   3. Maintain a low light level in the viewing area.
   A. 1 and 2
   B. 1 and 3
   C. 2 and 3
   D. 1, 2, and 3

3. When radiographs are viewed, the correct image orientation is:
   1. the way the anatomy was positioned when the image receptor (IR) was exposed.
   2. in the anatomic position.
   3. with the patient's right side toward the viewer's right side.
   A. 1 and 2
   B. 1 and 3
   C. 2 and 3
   D. 1, 2, and 3

4. The term *aesthetic quality* refers to the:
   A. visual appeal of the radiograph.
   B. position of the part on the IR.
   C. amount of detail in the image.
   D. amount of contrast in the image.

5. Images that lack aesthetic quality may:
   1. show artifacts.
   2. be too dark or too light.
   3. display poor alignment of the body part.
   A. 1 and 2
   B. 1 and 3
   C. 2 and 3
   D. 1, 2, and 3

6. Which of the following would be a factor used to evaluate evidence of radiation safety practices?
   A. Contrast
   B. Density
   C. Collimation
   D. Patient positioning

7. (True/False) The decision to repeat a radiograph should be based only on radiation safety considerations.

8. (True/False) Keeping a log of repeated radiographs aids the limited operator in evaluating problems and progressing toward aesthetic quality.

9. Troubleshooting an image includes:
   1. deciding whether the image should be repeated.
   2. determining the cause of any problems.
   3. discussing the image with the patient's physician.
   A. 1 and 2
   B. 1 and 3
   C. 2 and 3
   D. 1, 2, and 3

10. (True/False) Radiographs with markings added after exposure are not admissible in court.

11. (True/False) Errors in diagnosis can occur with incorrect position and exposure factors.

12. The factors that affect resolution include which of the following?
    1. Object–image receptor distance (OID)
    2. Motion
    3. Screen speed
    A. 1 and 2
    B. 1 and 3
    C. 2 and 3
    D. 1, 2, and 3

13. Which of the following will decrease patient motion in the radiograph?
    A. Use of low-mA (milliampere) techniques
    B. Use of low-kVp (peak kilovoltage) techniques
    C. Providing clear instructions
    D. Selection of a slow-speed screen if motion is anticipated

14. (True/False) The visual quality check for proper radiation exposure in digital radiography systems is to check the Exposure Indicator number.

191

15. Anatomic structures may be excluded in the image because of:
    1. inaccurate collimation.
    2. improper IR size.
    3. improper selection of mA or kVp.
    A. 1 and 2
    B. 1 and 3
    C. 2 and 3
    D. 1, 2, and 3

16. Radiographs of fingers, hands, toes, and feet are positioned on the viewing monitor with the:
    A. distal aspects pointing up.
    B. distal aspects pointing down.

17. A limited operator would be repeating radiographs unnecessarily if his or her repeat rate exceeded:
    A. 1%.
    B. 4%.
    C. 10%.
    D. 15%.

18. Most experienced limited operators have a repeat rate of about:
    A. 1%.
    B. 4%.
    C. 10%.
    D. 15%.

EXERCISE 2

Answer the following questions.

1. What is the acronym that can help you remember how to accurately assess image quality?

   _____

2. What does each letter stand for in the acronym that answers Question 1?

   Letter   Definition

   _____   _____

   _____   _____

   _____   _____

   _____   _____

   _____   _____

3. Describe the anatomic position.

   _____

   _____

   _____

   _____

   _____

CHALLENGE EXERCISE

This exercise does not have to be completed at the same time as the other exercises in this workbook chapter. The exercise is designed to assess retention of the essential information contained in the corresponding textbook chapter. In addition, many other chapters will need to be consulted to fully answer many of these questions, because image evaluation requires comprehensive understanding of imaging principles and procedural details. It is recommended that you complete this exercise when you begin to study for the state limited licensure examination. This will help determine what you know and which information should be further reviewed.

1. Describe the appearance of a screen-film radiograph that has been overexposed.

_____

2. Describe the appearance of a digital radiograph that has been overexposed.

_____

3. Describe the appearance of a screen-film radiograph that has been exposed with a kVp that was too low for the body part.

_____

4. Describe the appearance of a digital radiograph that has been exposed with a kVp that was too low for the body part.

_____

5. What is the most common cause of poor spatial resolution (detail) in a digital radiograph?

_____

6. Describe the appearance of a radiograph in which the OID of the part was too great.

_____

7. How could you correct the appearance of the radiograph in Question 6 if the OID of the part could not be decreased?

_____

8. Does central ray angulation result primarily in size distortion or shape distortion?

_____

9. Describe the correct placement of radiographic markers.

_____

_____

10. Describe the cause and appearance of noise on a radiograph.

_____

11. Because there is no direct link between exposure level and image brightness in digital radiographic systems, how do you determine whether a radiograph was taken with an appropriate exposure level?

_____

12. Describe radiation exposure conditions that will result in unsatisfactory digital images.

_____

_____

_____

20 Ethics, Legal Considerations, and Professionalism

EXERCISE 1

Answer the following questions.

1. List at least four characteristics that distinguish a profession from a nonprofessional occupation.

   1. _____

   2. _____

   3. _____

   4. _____

2. (True/False) Limited radiography is considered to be a profession.

3. (True/False) Professional attitudes and behaviors are expected of limited x-ray machine operators.

4. Define the following terms and give an example of each.

   1. Morals: _____

      _____

   2. Values: _____

      _____

   3. Ethics: _____

      _____

5. An aspirational document that establishes a high standard of professional conduct and assists the members of the radiologic technology profession in practicing ethical principles is the

   _____.

6. Mandatory standards of minimally acceptable professional conduct for all registered radiologic technologists are contained in the document called the

   _____.

   _____

7. Write a brief phrase that characterizes the behavior prescribed in each principle of the code of ethics of the American Registry of Radiologic Technologists.

Principle 1: _____

Principle 2: _____

Principle 3: _____

Principle 4: _____

Principle 5: _____

Principle 6: _____

Principle 7: _____

Principle 8: _____

Principle 9: _____

Principle 10: _____

8. (True/False) The confidentiality of conversations between patients and limited operators is not protected by "legal privilege."

9. (True/False) It is ethical to discuss your patients with your friends as long as you do not mention the patients' names.

10. List the four basic steps involved in solving ethical dilemmas using the process of ethical analysis.

   1. _____

   2. _____

   3. _____

   4. _____

EXERCISE 2

Answer the following questions.

1. (True/False) Most procedures commonly performed by limited operators require that the patient sign an informed consent document.

2. (True/False) Parents, grandparents, or adult siblings may sign an informed consent form for a minor.

3. (True/False) Informed consent may be revoked by the patient at any time after signing.

4. Explain briefly why it is essential to maintain all credentials that are required for practice.

_____

_____

_____

5. Match the types of intentional misconduct with their legal definitions.

1. _____ Assault   A. Unjustifiable detention

2. _____ Battery   B. Unlawful touching

3. _____ False imprisonment   C. Written information that causes defamation of character

4. _____ Invasion of privacy   D. Disclosure of confidential information

5. _____ Libel   E. Omission of reasonable care

6. _____ Slander   F. The threat of touching in an injurious way

                                                  G. Verbal dissemination of information that causes loss of reputation

6. Failure to use reasonable care or caution is termed _____.

7. What is the standard of care that is used to legally define negligence?

_____

8. The responsibility of health care providers for accountability in the area of patient confidentiality is legally pre-

scribed in a federal law known by the acronym _____.

9. An act of negligence in the context of a professional relationship is defined as professional negligence or

_____

10. The employer is liable for employees' negligent acts that occur in the course of their work, according to the legal

doctrine of _____.

11. List three important steps you can take to reduce the likelihood of malpractice litigation.

1. _____

2. _____

3. _____

EXERCISE 3

Answer the following questions.

1. Number the following list of human needs in order according to the hierarchy of needs, with 1 being the most basic level of needs and 6 being the highest level.

_____ Love and acceptance   _____ Recreation

_____ Nutrition and oxygen   _____ Self-actualization

_____ Recognition   _____ Safety

                                  Chapter **20** **Ethics, Legal Considerations, and Professionalism**

2. List good practices that represent responsible self-care by limited operators.

_____

_____

_____

_____

_____

3. List three positive actions for promoting teamwork and cooperation in the workplace.

1. _____

2. _____

3. _____

4. Sensitivity to the needs of others that allows you to meet those needs constructively is called

_____.

5. What is the best strategy for dealing with clinical situations in which you find it difficult to cope because the patient is vomiting, bleeding, or acting inappropriately?

_____

6. List reasons why limited operators should pursue continuing education, even if it is not required for the renewal of credentials.

_____

_____

_____

EXERCISE 4

Answer the following questions.

1. List three nonverbal behaviors that enhance communication.

1. _____

2. _____

3. _____

2. Explain what is meant by *validation of communication.*

_____

_____

3. List three useful strategies for successful communication under stress.

  1. _____

  2. _____

  3. _____

4. Write two questions other than those presented in the text that could be used to offer an adult patient a valid choice.

  1. _____

  2. _____

5. Match the following communication terms with the correct definitions.

  1. _____ Validation   A. Sensitivity to the needs of others

  2. _____ Aggression   B. Reaction to the distress of others

  3. _____ Empathy   C. Calm, firm expression of feelings or opinions

  4. _____ Assertion   D. Confirmation that a message is understood

  5. _____ Sympathy   E. Expression of angry or hostile feelings

                                         F. Disregard for the feelings of others

EXERCISE 5

Answer the following questions.

  1. List signs or characteristics that might alert you to the fact that a patient is totally deaf.

  _____

  _____

  _____

  _____

  2. List three ways in which the deaf may communicate.

  1. _____

  2. _____

  3. _____

  3. (True/False) Patients who do not speak English are responsible for communicating effectively in a health care situation despite language barriers.

  4. (True/False) When patients do not speak English, translation by a family member is preferable to translation by an interpreter who is not known by the patient.

Chapter **20** **Ethics, Legal Considerations, and Professionalism**

5. (True/False) When using an interpreter, you should talk directly to the patient as if he or she could understand you.

6. List common social practices in the United States that might be different in other cultures.

_____

_____

_____

7. An old superstition of Mediterranean origin that is occasionally seen among Hispanic patients is called the *evil eye,* or *mal ojo.* This is a belief that _____

_____

8. Check the cultural groups listed below in which direct eye contact is generally acceptable.

_____ Many cultures in the United States

_____ Most Asian cultures

_____ Native American cultures

_____ Hispanic culture

_____ Russian culture

9. Aggressive demands for service and attention by patients' families are most commonly results of _____

_____.

10. List three things you can do to support the anxious relatives of an injured patient.

1. _____

2. _____

3. _____

EXERCISE 6

Answer the following questions.

1. A legal document that contains a record of the care and treatment received by a patient is called a _____

_____.

2. Diagnostic images are owned by _____

_____.

3. What should you do if a physician calls from across town and requests images that are in your files?

_____

_____

CHALLENGE EXERCISE

This exercise does not have to be completed at the same time as the other exercises in this workbook chapter. The exercise is designed to assess retention of the essential information contained in the corresponding textbook chapter. It is recommended that you complete this exercise when you begin to study for the state limited licensure examination. This will help determine what you know and which information should be further reviewed.

1. What constitutes a medical chart?

_____

_____

2. Who owns diagnostic images?

_____

3. Who bears responsibility for communication when a patient is unable to speak or understand English?

_____

4. *Negligence* is defined as failure to use reasonable care or caution. How is this standard defined?

_____

5. The use of physical restraints without the patient's permission or a physician's order could be the basis for a legal charge of _____.

6. Failure to maintain confidence in a clinical situation could result in a legal charge of _____

_____.

7. What is the ethical responsibility of a limited operator with respect to the diagnosis or interpretation of images?

_____

8. A limited operator should not discriminate against any patient on the basis of gender, age, race, ethnicity, or diagnosis. Such discrimination is a violation of _____.

9. When the solution to a problem is sought through a process that includes identification of the problem, development of alternate solutions, selecting the best solution, and defending the selection, this process is called

_____.

10. The aspirational document that establishes ethical standards for those involved in medical imaging is _____

_____.

21 Safety and Infection Control

EXERCISE 1

Answer the following questions.

1. In the list below, check the three elements that must be present in order for a fire to burn.

    _____ Open flames

    _____ Fuel

    _____ Smoke

    _____ Oxygen

    _____ Electricity

    _____ Heat

2. (True/False) In case of an electrical fire, you should use a class A fire extinguisher or a water supply to put out the fire.

3. (True/False) Oxygen does not burn.

4. List three important fire safety precautions that should be observed when oxygen is in use.

    1. _____

    2. _____

    3. _____

5. What should you know about a clinical facility to be prepared in case of fire?

    _____

    _____

    _____

6. Give the acronym for remembering the four basic steps to follow in case of fire. Write the meaning of each letter in the acronym.

    _____

    _____

    _____

    _____

8. Padding should be placed under bony prominences such as the sacrum, heels, or midthoracic curvature of older or debilitated patients for comfort and to prevent the development of _____.

9. When assisting a patient to lie down, place one arm _____ and the other

_____.

10. It is preferable for patients suffering from recent back injuries and those recovering from spinal surgery to sit up from

the _____ position.

11. A temporary state of low blood pressure that causes patients to feel light-headed or faint when they first sit up is

termed _____.

12. *(Circle the correct phrase.)* When assisting a patient who has weakness on one side of the body to walk, position yourself on the patient's (strong side/weak side).

13. The most common type of fall associated with wheelchair transfer occurs when _____

_____.

14. (True/False) The use of sandbags to immobilize trembling extremities can assist in minimizing motion, even when the area of interest does not involve the extremity.

15. (True/False) The application of physical restraints to the arms or legs of an adult patient without the patient's consent requires a physician's order.

16. (True/False) An incident report must be completed only for occurrences that result in injury to a patient.

EXERCISE 3

Answer the following questions.

1. The four principal factors involved in the spread of disease, sometimes called the *cycle of infection,* are:

    1. _____

    2. _____

    3. _____

    4. _____

2. Match the following terms referring to microorganisms and other infectious agents with their definitions.

1. _____ Normal flora   A. The smallest and least understood of all infectious agents

2. _____ Pathogens   B. Very small subcellular organisms such as those that cause influenza, chickenpox, and the common cold

3. _____ Bacteria

     C. Bacterial forms that are resistant to heat, cold, and drying and can live without nourishment

4. _____ Viruses

     D. Agents that cause disease

5. _____ Endospores

     E. Complex single-cell animals that generally exist as free-living organisms

6. _____ Fungi

     F. Microorganisms that live on or within the body without causing disease

7. _____ Prions

     G. Very small single-cell organisms with a cell wall and an atypical nucleus that lacks a

8. _____ Protozoa   membrane; named for their shapes, including bacilli, cocci, spirochetes, and spirilla

     H. Occur as single-celled yeasts or as filament-like structures called molds

3. Describe the five indirect routes of disease transmission, and give an example of each.

    1. Fomite: _____

_____

    2. Vector: _____

_____

    3. Vehicle: _____

_____

    4. Airborne contamination: _____

_____

    5. Droplet contamination: _____

_____

4. The agency that monitors and studies the types of infections occurring in the United States and compiles and publishes statistical data about these infections is _____.

5. The infectious agent that causes acquired immunodeficiency syndrome (AIDS) is _____

_____.

6. In the list below, check the types of contact that may result in the transmission of human immunodeficiency virus (HIV).

_____ Shaking hands   _____ Sharing contaminated needles

_____ Sexual intercourse   _____ Contact with drinking fountains

_____ Eating food prepared by an infected individual   _____ Contact with toilets

7. (True/False) There is no known cure for AIDS.

8. (True/False) The patient's right to confidentiality regarding AIDS diagnosis or HIV status may prevent you from being informed about the patient's status.

9. (True/False) There are thousands of documented, confirmed cases of HIV infection in health care workers resulting from accidental needlesticks.

10. The hepatitis B virus (HBV) is spread through contact with _____.

11. The types of hepatitis that are spread through contact with food or water contaminated with feces are type _____

_____ and type _____.

12. Vaccine is available to protect health care workers from infection by which hepatitis virus? _____

_____.

13. If postexposure prophylaxis (PEP) is recommended following a needlestick injury, how soon after the injury should

this therapy be administered? _____

14. Pulmonary tuberculosis is spread by means of _____

_____.

15. (True/False) Most of those who become infected with tubercle bacilli develop a clinical disease and become infectious to others.

16. (True/False) Lowered resistance because of immunodeficiency, malnutrition, other illness, or old age may cause reactivation of a tuberculosis infection.

17. The simplest and most common method of testing for tuberculosis infection is the _____

_____.

18. The standard precautions defined by the Centers for Disease Control and Prevention (CDC) call for the use of barriers whenever contact is anticipated with four things, which are:

   1. _____

   2. _____

   3. _____

   4. _____

19. List three pathogens that are commonly responsible for health care–associated infections (HAIs).

   1. _____

   2. _____

   3. _____

EXERCISE 4

Answer the following questions.

1. The destruction of pathogens by chemical agents is called _____.

2. Treating items with heat, gas, or chemicals to make them germ free is called _____.

3. Decontamination of the hands using soap and water, an antiseptic hand wash, or an alcohol-based hand rub is called

   _____.

4. (True/False) Alcohol hand rubs are effective against most microorganisms.

5. (True/False) Hand hygiene is not necessary when gloves are worn.

6. When should washing with soap and water be used for hand hygiene instead of an alcohol rub? _____

   _____

7. As a cleaning agent for decontaminating environmental surfaces, the CDC recommends either a disinfectant registered by the Environmental Protection Agency as effective against HIV, HBV, and the tuberculosis bacterium or ____

   _____.

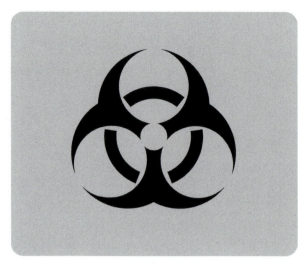

FIG. 21.2 Symbol.

8. Fig. 21.2 is a symbol that indicates _____.

9. (True/False) You should not remove anything from a hazardous waste container once it has been placed inside.

10. (True/False) To prevent needlestick injuries, you should always recap needles.

11. A receptacle for the disposal of needles, syringes, and contaminated items capable of puncturing the skin is called a

_____.

12. The quickest and most convenient means of sterilization for items that can withstand heat is _____

_____.

13. The type of sterilization that is used for telephones, stethoscopes, blood pressure cuffs, and other equipment that can-

not withstand heat is _____.

14. A germ-free area prepared for the use of sterile supplies and equipment is called a _____

_____.

15. The first step in preparing a sterile field is to confirm the sterility of packaged supplies and equipment. List the criteria that indicate when packages are considered sterile.

1. _____

2. _____

3. _____

16. *(Circle the correct phrase.)* When opening a sterile pack, open the first corner (toward you/away from you).

17. (True/False) It is all right to reach across a sterile field as long as you do not touch anything that is sterile.

18. (True/False) Any sterile object or field touched by an unsterile object or person becomes contaminated.

19. (True/False) Before adding a liquid to a sterile tray, you should discard a small amount from the container to rinse the container's lip.

20. *(Circle the correct word.)* The (application/removal) of a dressing is a procedure that requires sterile technique.

CHALLENGE EXERCISE

This exercise does not have to be completed at the same time as the other exercises in this workbook chapter. The exercise is designed to assess retention of the essential information contained in the corresponding textbook chapter. It is recommended that you complete this exercise when you begin to study for the state limited licensure examination. This will help determine what you know and which information should be further reviewed.

1. Why is it important to observe special fire safety precautions in areas where oxygen is in use?

   _____

2. What is the name of the position in which a patient is recumbent on the left lateral aspect of the body with the right

   knee flexed? _____

3. What is the name of the position in which a patient is supine with the head lower than the feet?

   _____

4. Orthopnea is a condition in which _____.

5. Microorganisms that cause disease are termed _____.

6. When assisting a patient to walk who has weakness on one side of the body, on which side should you position your-

   self? _____

7. Name a disease that requires the use of personal respirator equipment, isolation rooms with negative air pressure and

   special ventilation or circulation, and annual training about the disease. _____

   How is this disease transmitted? _____

8. Name the two principal means by which the human immunodeficiency virus is spread.

   _____

   _____

9. The CDC recommends a system of infection control that calls for the use of barriers whenever contact with blood,

   body fluids, or mucous membranes is anticipated. This system is called _____

   _____

10. Under what circumstances is the use of an alcohol hand rub an inadequate form of hand hygiene?

    _____

22 Assessing Patients and Managing Acute Situations

EXERCISE 1

Answer the following questions.

1. List the three skills that will help you adequately determine patients' needs.

   1. _____

   2. _____

   3. _____

2. List steps you can take to reassure and comfort patients who feel anxious.

   _____

   _____

   _____

3. List considerations that might help meet patients' physiologic needs.

   _____

   _____

4. Loss of bladder control is termed _____.

5. List the six characteristics of a patient's chief complaint that should be addressed in the questions used to elicit a preliminary medical history of the complaint.

   1. _____

   2. _____

   3. _____

   4. _____

   5. _____

   6. _____

EXERCISE 2

Answer the following questions.

1. When a patient exhibits a bluish coloration in the mucous membranes of the lips and in the nail beds, the patient

   is said to be _____.

2. When a patient is described as diaphoretic, this means that the patient is _____.

3. Hot, dry skin may indicate that the patient has _____.

4. *(Circle the correct word.)* Rectal temperatures are (higher/lower) than oral temperatures.

5. *(Circle the correct word.)* Axillary temperatures are (higher/lower) than oral temperatures.

6. When is it *not* appropriate to take a patient's temperature orally?

   _____

   _____

7. A rapid pulse, when the heart beats more than 100 times per minute, is called _____.

8. A pulse that is described as thready is one that is both _____ and _____.

9. *(Circle the correct word.)* The first or upper number in a blood pressure value is the (diastolic/systolic) pressure.

10. *(Circle the correct word.)* The term *hypertension* refers to (high/low) blood pressure.

11. The cuff and gauge for measuring blood pressure are called a(n):

    A. stethoscope.

    B. sphygmomanometer.

    C. tympanic thermometer.

    D. aneroid barometer.

12. List two steps you should take to ensure that emergency supplies are ready for use when an emergency arises.

    1. _____

    2. _____

EXERCISE 3

Answer the following questions.

1. *(Circle the correct term.)* In an emergency situation, oxygen is usually administered by means of a (mask/nasal cannula).

2. The usual flow rate for oxygen administration by face mask is _____.

3. *(Circle the correct word.)* Patients suffering from emphysema should receive an oxygen flow rate that is (greater/less) than the usual or average rate.

4. When a patient is unable to swallow or to cope with secretions, blood, or vomitus, you should prepare to assist with

   _____.

5. If a patient complains of sudden, intense pain under the sternum, you should assume until proved otherwise that the

   patient might be having _____.

EXERCISE 4

Answer the following questions.

1. When a patient suddenly loses consciousness, the first thing you should do is _____

    _____.

2. Lack of effective circulation to the central nervous system for five minutes can cause _____

    _____.

3. A rapid, weak, and ineffective heartbeat caused by interruption of the electric signals that control the heart is called

    _____.

4. When bleeding or swelling occurs inside the skull, seizures, loss of consciousness, or respiratory arrest may occur

    because of increased _____.

5. When a blow to the head causes damage on the side of the head opposite the side of the blow, this is termed a

    _____.

6. List the four levels of consciousness.

    1. _____

    2. _____

    3. _____

    4. _____

7. A fracture in which the bone protrudes through the skin is called a _____.

8. Continuous, abnormal blood flow is called _____.

9. Redness of the skin is termed _____.

10. A severe allergic reaction is termed _____ or _____.

11. An antihistamine medication, such as diphenhydramine, may be given as a treatment for _____

    _____.

12. Anaphylaxis is a type of shock caused by _____.

13. An individual who is terribly thirsty, urinates copious amounts frequently, and has fruity-smelling breath may be

    approaching a state of _____.

14. An enzyme normally produced in the pancreas that aids in the digestion of glucose is _____.

15. A cerebrovascular accident (CVA) is also called a _____.

23 Medications and Their Administration

Answer the following questions.

1. List duties related to medication administration that a limited operator may perform, even if not permitted to actually administer the medication.

   1. _____

   2. _____

   3. _____

   4. _____

   5. _____

2. Whose duty is it to determine the route of administration for a medication? _____

3. (True/False) A standing order might allow a nurse to administer a specific dose of nitroglycerin to a patient experiencing angina when the physician is not present.

4. (True/False) Checking expiration dates on medication supplies is not important in physicians' offices and clinics, because such supplies are used infrequently.

5. The name of a drug that identifies its specific chemical composition is called its _____.

6. The brand name given to a product by its manufacturer is called its _____ or

   _____ name.

7. Match the following types of medication effects with their definitions.

   1. _____ Toxic   A. Produces a specific action that promotes a desired effect

   2. _____ Agonistic   B. Causes an unusual or peculiar effect, or the opposite of the expected effect

   3. _____ Antagonistic   C. Effect of two or more drugs whose combined effect is beyond the individual effects
                                of each drug alone

   4. _____ Synergistic
                             D. Has poisonous consequences

   5. _____ Idiosyncratic
                             E. Prevents or reverses the effects of other drugs

8. The government agency that sets standards for the control of drugs is the _____.

9. The efficacy of a drug refers to its _____.

10. The potency of a drug refers to its _____.

Answer the following questions.

1. Match the following routes of administration with their definitions.

   1. _____ Topical   A. Inside the cheek

   2. _____ Intradermal   B. Under the skin

   3. _____ Intramuscular   C. Between the skin layers

   4. _____ Sublingual   D. Within a vein

   5. _____ Buccal   E. Under the tongue

   6. _____ Subcutaneous   F. Within the muscle

   7. _____ Intravenous   G. By mouth, swallowed

   8. _____ Oral   H. On the skin

2. Match the following drug classes with their applications.

   1. _____ Antihistamine   A. Antimicrobial, prevents or treats infection

   2. _____ Antibiotic   B. Antiinflammatory, treats inflammation, including that caused by allergic
                                  reactions

   3. _____ NSAID
                               C. Tranquilizer, sedates

   4. _____ Anesthetic
                               D. Analgesic, relieves pain

   5. _____ Corticosteroid
                               E. Antiallergic, relieves symptoms of allergic reactions

   6. _____ Benzodiazepine
                               F. Eliminates sensation

3. Medication effect is determined to some degree by the water content of body tissues, which is termed _____

   _____.

4. Match the following terms related to pharmacokinetics with their definitions.

   1. _____ Excretion   A. The process by which the body transforms drugs into an inactive form that can
                                  be eliminated from the body

   2. _____ Absorption
                               B. The process by which the drug enters the systemic circulation to provide a

   3. _____ Metabolism   desired effect

   4. _____ Distribution   C. The elimination of drugs from the body

                               D. The means by which drugs travel to the site of action

5. The most common mechanism of drug action is the binding of drugs to _____

   _____.

6. Drugs are administered to produce a predictable physiologic response called the _____

_____ .

7. Opioids and other substances whose availability is strictly regulated or outlawed because of their potential for abuse or

addiction are called _____ substances.

8. Life-threatening respiratory depression is a possible side effect following the administration of _____

_____ .

9. A specific drug that treats a toxic effect is called a(n) _____ .

EXERCISE 3

Answer the following questions.

1. If a child weighs 30 pounds, what is the child's weight in kilograms? _____

2. If a drug is supplied in a strength of 5 mg/mL, and you want to administer 15 mg, you will need _____ mL.

3. If 5 mL of a drug has been administered and the strength is 30 mcg/mL, what dose was given?

_____

4. (True/False) The Occupational Safety and Health Administration regulations now require the use of engineering controls to decrease the risk to health care workers from contaminated needlesticks.

5. (True/False) A 22-gauge needle is larger around than an 18-gauge needle and delivers a given volume of fluid more rapidly.

6. For intramuscular injection in small children, the preferred muscle site is the _____ .

7. The height of the bottle or bag used for intravenous infusion affects the flow rate and should always be _____

_____ inches above the level of the vein.

8. When the area around an intravenous infusion injection site is cool, swollen, and boggy, these are signs that:

_____

9. When extravasation occurs during an intravenous injection or infusion, you should _____

_____

10. (True/False) You should wear protective gloves when giving injections.

11. (True/False) Aseptic technique should always be followed for injection procedures.

12. List the information that must be included when the administration of a medication is charted.

_____

_____

_____

24 Medical Laboratory Skills

EXERCISE 1

Answer the following questions.

1. Standard precautions were developed to protect health care workers from infection with

   _____.

2. The essence of standard precautions is embodied in the statement that

   _____.

3. List the three essential aspects of the standard precautions as they relate to handling blood and urine.

   1. _____

   2. _____

   3. _____

4. Any refuse that is poisonous or dangerous to living creatures is termed.

   _____.

5. Objects that can puncture the skin, such as needles, glass tubes, glass slides, and finger lancets, must be disposed of in a(n)

   _____.

EXERCISE 2

Answer the following questions.

1. The technique of entering a vein with a needle to withdraw a blood sample is termed

   _____.

2. The veins most commonly used for obtaining blood samples are located in the

   _____.

3. The evacuated plastic tubes used for blood specimen collection have color-coded stoppers that indicate

   _____.

4. List two ways in which the handling of blood specimen tubes that have additives differs from the handling of those that do not.

   1. _____

   2. _____

5. (True/False) An evacuated blood specimen tube cannot be used a second time following an unsuccessful venipuncture.

6. State the needle gauge and length for routine venipuncture:

   _____ gauge, _____ inches in length.

7. A standard venipuncture needle is actually two needles attached to a threaded plastic hub. The needle mounted

   to the threaded side of the hub is designed to puncture _____. The other

   needle, mounted to the nonthreaded end of the hub, is for puncturing _____.

8. (True/False) Special venipuncture needles with engineered sharps injury protection are available to minimize the risk of needlestick injury to personnel and to comply with the requirements of the Occupational Safety and Health Administration.

9. (True/False) Venipuncture needle holders (barrels) are reusable items.

10. A tight band placed around the arm to facilitate distention of the vein for venipuncture is called a(n)

    _____

11. Alcohol preparation wipes are generally used to cleanse the skin for venipuncture, but povidone–iodine wipes must

    be used if the specimen is being collected for _____ or _____

    _____

12. (True/False) Some manufacturers produce evacuated tubes with stoppers covered by plastic caps to minimize aerosol production; these caps eliminate the need to use a shield when opening specimen tubes.

13. List three sites that should be avoided when selecting a site for venipuncture.

    1. _____

    2. _____

    3. _____

14. Choice of a vein for venipuncture is based on _____.

15. (Circle the correct word.) When obtaining a blood specimen, you should engage the vacuum tube on the internal needle (before/after) the external needle is properly situated in the vein.

16. (Circle the correct word.) When all blood specimens have been obtained, you should remove the last tube from the needle holder (before/after) removing the needle from the vein.

17. Failure of the tube to fill with blood during venipuncture means that _____

    _____.

EXERCISE 3

Answer the following questions.

1. The physical, microscopic, and/or chemical examination of urine is termed _____.

2. List the three components of a routine urinalysis.

    1. _____

    2. _____

    3. _____

3. What should you do to maintain the quality and accuracy of reagent strips?

    _____

    _____

4. (True/False) *Urinalysis tube* is another term for a urine specimen collection cup.

5. When should a urine specimen be collected to obtain the greatest amount of diagnostic information?

    _____

6. Urine collected regardless of the time of day is termed a(n)_____.

7. The correct method for collecting a urine specimen is called the _____.

8. *(Circle the correct phrase.)* When a female cleanses the labia for a clean-catch midstream specimen, the cleansing sponge or towelette is wiped in a(n) (anterior to posterior/posterior to anterior) direction.

9. If a urine specimen cannot be analyzed promptly, how should the specimen be handled when first obtained and before analysis?

    _____

    _____

    _____

10. List the two characteristics to be assessed in a macroscopic (visual) examination of urine.

    1. _____

    2. _____

11. (True/False) When a urine reagent strip is read, timing is critical, and the test result must be read in the time indicated by the manufacturer.

12. When the color of a urine reagent strip does not match any of the reference colors and the test has been repeated with the same results using a strip from a different bottle, what should you do?

    _____

3. Describe the attenuation method used in BMD calculation.

_____

_____

_____

_____

4. Why is a baseline scan so important in diagnosis and follow-up?

_____

_____

5. How often should you perform a phantom scan?

_____

_____

6. Name one contraindication to performing a central DXA scan.

_____

_____

7. Describe the difference between accuracy and precision in bone densitometry.

_____

_____

8. What does ALARA stand for?

_____

9. What is the minimal distance a DXA operator should be from the x-ray source of a fan-beam DXA scanner?

_____

10. Define the difference between primary and secondary osteoporosis.

_____

_____

_____

_____

11. What is the correct procedure to follow after there has been a failed quality assurance test on any DXA scanner?

_____

_____

_____

_____

_____

12. Describe FRAX and why it is used.

_____

_____

13. What is the primary reason a serial DXA scan is done?

_____

_____

B. Describe the steps the operator must take to ensure proper comparison with the baseline lumbar spine scan.

_____

_____

_____

_____

_____

_____

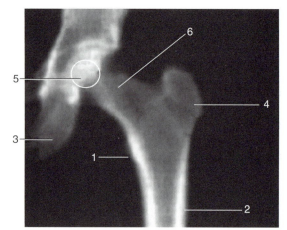

FIG. 26.3 Image of femur. (Courtesy of Erickson Retirement Bone Health Program, 2008.)

3. Match the following parts of this proximal femur image with the corresponding number.

Greater trochanter   _____

Femoral neck   _____

Femoral head   _____

Pelvic ischium   _____

Lesser trochanter   _____

Femoral shaft   _____

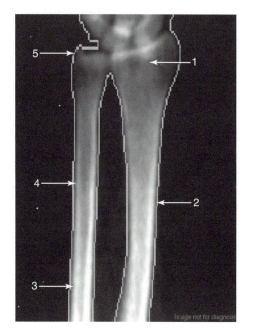

FIG. 26.4 Anatomy of the forearm. (Courtesy of Erickson Retirement Bone Health Program, 2008.)

4. Match the following parts of this forearm image with the corresponding number.

Ulna   _____

Radius   _____

Distal radius   _____

Proximal ulna   _____

Ulnar styloid   _____

SECTION TWO   PREPARATION GUIDE FOR THE AMERICAN REGISTRY OF RADIOLOGIC TECHNOLOGISTS EXAMINATION FOR THE LIMITED SCOPE OF PRACTICE IN RADIOGRAPHY

Introduction

This guide is provided to help you prepare to successfully complete the licensure examination for the limited scope of practice area in which you are or will be working. We have included helpful suggestions for optimizing your study time and a simulated examination to help you identify your areas of strength and weakness. All suggestions and discussions are based on the American Registry of Radiologic Technologists (ARRT) Content Specifications for the Examination for the Limited Scope of Practice in Radiography. We have done this for two reasons: first, this is a comprehensive examination covering all relevant areas of practice, and second, it is likely that the licensure agency in your state uses this examination. If your state does not use this examination, you will still be well prepared if you use the ARRT Content Specifications as your study guide. For your convenience, we have included the most recent ARRT Content Specifications in this guide.

If you are using *Radiography Essentials for Limited Practice* and this accompanying workbook, it is likely that you are participating in an educational program designed to prepare you both to work in a given practice area and to successfully pass the appropriate state licensure examination. This guide should assist you in both these endeavors. Completing the simulated examination will help you identify knowledge that you have already acquired and knowledge that you have yet to master. Because the simulated examination was constructed to assess content identified in the ARRT Content Specifications, it is appropriate to provide an overview of the latter document before moving on to the examination.

The ARRT Content Specifications for the Examination for the Limited Scope of Practice in Radiography covers five practice areas by administering five radiographic procedure modules. These include the chest, extremities, skull and sinuses, spine, and podiatric. The ARRT Content Specifications indicate that there are two components to each practice area licensure examination: a core module that everyone completes and one or more radiographic procedure modules. The core module assesses knowledge in the areas of radiation protection, equipment operation and quality control, image production and evaluation, and patient care and education. According to the Content Specifications document, the ARRT believes

that all individuals licensed in limited scope radiography should know this information. Which of the radiographic procedure modules you take will depend on your area of practice. If your practice area is limited to chest radiography, you will complete only the chest module. However, if there is a licensure category in your state that allows radiography in all the procedural areas, you will complete all five modules. Licensure laws differ by state, and each licensure agency has its own procedures and guidelines.

The most valuable component of the AART Content Specifications is the outline of each content area covered on the examination. The numbers in parentheses in this outline indicate how many questions on the examination assess some aspect of knowledge in the designated area. The value to you is that this information will help you determine how much time and effort to spend on certain topics. Without using this information as a guide, you may waste valuable time learning information that is not included on the examination. However, we are not suggesting that you deviate from the curriculum established by your state agency or by your teacher. This guide is to help you prepare for the state licensure examination, not to prepare you to work in your practice area. You will need skills that cannot be directly assessed by a written examination.

The limited scope simulated examination is located after the ARRT Content Specifications in this section. You will find a core module and five radiographic procedure modules. You should complete the core module portion of the examination, regardless of your practice area. After completing the core module, complete the module or modules appropriate for your practice area. You should schedule time to complete all relevant portions of the examination at the same time. This will give you experience in completing an examination of that length and give you some idea of how long it will take you to do so.

The core module consists of 100 questions, as prescribed in the ARRT Content Specifications, and contains the appropriate number of questions from each of the four content areas: radiation protection (37), equipment operation and quality control (11), image production and evaluation (35), and patient care and education (17). The questions are further focused to cover content specified in

241

Introduction

the outline for each content area. You will see that there are more content topics in each outline than there are questions included in the examination. This means that some content will not be assessed with a question, both on the simulated examination and on your actual state licensure examination. That is why it is important for you to review all topics included in each content outline in the ARRT Content Specifications. You cannot rely only on the simulated examination to prepare you for your state licensure examination.

The five radiographic procedure modules are located after the core module. Each contains the appropriate number of questions prescribed in the ARRT Content Specifications for the five modules: chest (20), extremities (25), skull and sinuses (20), spine (25), and podiatric (20) radiography. The questions are further focused to cover content specified in the outline for each module. As mentioned in the previous paragraph, there are more content topics in each outline than are questions included in the examination. Therefore, some content will not be assessed with a question, both on the simulated examination and on your actual state licensure examination. For this reason, you should review all topics included in each content outline in the ARRT Content Specifications.

The answers to all simulated examination questions in each examination module are located after the last question in the module. We have included the correct answer (ANS), as well as the textbook chapter in *Radiography*

Essentials for Limited Practice in which the information is located (REF), the designator for the ARRT Content Specifications topic outline item (OBJ) that the question is designed to assess, and the topic (TOP) addressed by the question. This information will allow you to easily find and review text material that you have not yet mastered.

Your timeline to prepare for the state licensure examination should be something like the following:

Participate in the educational program.
- Complete all workbook exercises related to the given area of practice. Do not waste time on radiographic procedures chapters outside your licensure area. This activity is especially important if you are not in a formal education program.
- Complete all Challenge Exercises at the end of each relevant workbook chapter.
- Complete the simulated examination.
- Analyze the results of your examination to identify information you have not yet mastered.
- Review information related to questions you missed on the examination. It may be helpful to repeat relevant workbook exercises.
- Complete the simulated examination again and analyze the results. Review additional information as needed.
- Successfully complete the state limited scope licensure examination!

ARRT Content Specifications for the Limited Scope of Practice in Radiography Examination

CONTENT SPECIFICATIONS FOR THE LIMITED SCOPE OF PRACTICE IN RADIOGRAPHY EXAMINATION

ARRT Board Approved: January 2014
Implementation Date: January 2015

The purpose of the Limited Scope of Practice in Radiography Examination, which is developed and administered by The American Registry of Radiologic Technologists® (ARRT®) on behalf of state licensing agencies, is to assess the knowledge and cognitive skills underlying the intelligent performance of the tasks typically required of operators of radiographic equipment used to radiograph selected anatomic regions (chest, extremities, etc.). ARRT administers the examination to state approved candidates under contractual arrangement with the state and provides the results directly to the state. This examination is not associated with any type of certification by the ARRT.

The knowledge and skills covered by the examination were determined by administering a comprehensive practice analysis survey to a nationwide sample of radiographers and adopting a subset of the tasks developed for the radiography task inventory as the limited scope task inventory. The task inventory appears in Attachment D of this document. The content specifications for the limited scope examination identify the knowledge areas underlying performance of the tasks on the limited scope task inventory. Every content category can be linked to one or more activities on the task inventory.

It is the philosophy of the ARRT that an individual licensed in limited scope radiography possess the same knowledge and cognitive skill, in his or her specific area of radiography, as radiographers. The modules covered by the examination are outlined below. Subsequent pages describe in detail the topics covered within each module. All candidates take the CORE module of the examination and one or more RADIOGRAPHIC PROCEDURE modules, depending on the type of license for which they have applied.

Core Module		Number of Scored Questions[1]	Testing Time
A.	Radiation Protection	37	
B.	Equipment Operation and Quality Control	11	
C.	Image Acquisition and Evaluation	35	
D.	Patient Care and Education	17	
	Total for Core Module	100	1 hr, 55 min

E. Radiographic Procedure Modules

E.1	Chest	20	20 min
E.2	Extremities	25	25 min
E.3	Skull/Sinuses	20	20 min
E.4	Spine	25	25 min
E.5	Podiatric	20	25 min

[1]The core module includes an additional 15 unscored (pilot) questions. Each of the radiographic procedure modules has five additional unscored questions.

Copyright © 2014 by The American Registry of Radiologic Technologists.

243

A. RADIATION PROTECTION (37)

1. **Biologic Aspects of Radiation (7)**
   A. Radiosensitivity
      1. dose-response relationships
      2. relative tissue radiosensitivities (e.g., LET, RBE)
      3. cell survival and recovery (LD_{50})
      4. oxygen effect
   B. Somatic Effects
      1. short-term versus long-term effects
      2. acute versus chronic effects
      3. carcinogenesis
      4. organ and tissue response (e.g., eye, thyroid, breast, bone marrow, skin, gonadal)
   C. Acute Radiation Syndromes
      1. CNS
      2. hemopoietic
      3. GI
   D. Embryonic and Fetal Risks
   E. Genetic Impact
      1. genetic significant dose
      2. goals of gonadal shielding
   F. Photon Interactions with Matter
      1. Compton effect
      2. photoelectric absorption
      3. coherent (classical) scatter
      4. attenuation by various tissues
         a. thickness of body part (density)
         b. type of tissue (atomic number)

2. **Minimizing Patient Exposure (13)**
   A. Exposure Factors
      1. kVp
      2. mAs
   B. Shielding
      1. rationale for use
      2. types
      3. placement
   C. Beam Restriction
      1. purpose of primary beam restriction
      2. types (e.g., collimators)
   D. Filtration
      1. effect on skin and organ exposure
      2. effect on average beam energy
      3. NCRP recommendations (NCRP #102, minimum filtration in useful beam)

   E. Exposure Reduction
      1. patient positioning
      2. patient communication
      3. digital imaging
      4. pediatric dose reduction
      5. ALARA
   F. Image Receptors (e.g., types, relative speed, digital versus film)

3. **Personnel Protection (9)**
   A. Sources of Radiation Exposure
      1. primary x-ray beam
      2. secondary radiation
         a. scatter
         b. leakage
      3. patient as source
   B. Basic Methods of Protection
      1. time
      2. distance
      3. shielding
   C. Protective Devices
      1. types
      2. attenuation properties
      3. minimum lead equivalent (NCRP #102)

4. **Radiation Exposure and Monitoring (8)**
   A. Units of Measurement*
      1. absorbed dose
      2. dose equivalent
      3. exposure
   B. Dosimeters
      1. types
      2. proper use
   C. NCRP Recommendations for Personnel Monitoring (NCRP #116)
      1. occupational exposure
      2. public exposure
      3. embryo/fetus exposure
      4. ALARA and dose equivalent limits
      5. evaluation and maintenance of personnel dosimetry records

---

*Conventional units are generally used. However, questions referenced to specific reports (e.g., NCRP) will use SI units to be consistent with such reports.

B. EQUIPMENT OPERATION AND QUALITY CONTROL (11)

1. **Principles of Radiation Physics (3)**
   A. X-Ray Production
      1. source of free electrons (e.g., thermionic emission)
      2. acceleration of electrons
      3. focusing of electrons
      4. deceleration of electrons
   B. Target Interactions
      1. bremsstrahlung
      2. characteristic
   C. X-Ray Beam
      1. frequency and wavelength
      2. beam characteristics
         a. quality
         b. quantity
         c. primary versus remnant (exit)
      3. inverse square law
      4. fundamental properties (e.g., travel in straight lines, ionize matter)

2. **Imaging Equipment (4)**
   A. Components of Radiographic Unit (fixed or mobile)
      1. operating console
      2. x-ray tube construction
         a. electron sources
         b. target materials
         c. induction motor
      3. manual exposure controls
      4. beam restriction devices
   B. X-Ray Generator, Transformers, and Rectification System (basic principles)
   C. Components of Digital Imaging (CR and DR)
      1. PSP—photo-stimulable phosphor
      2. flat panel detectors—direct and indirect
      3. CR reader components
      4. CR plate erasure
      5. equipment cleanliness (imaging plates, CR plates)

3. **Quality Control of Imaging Equipment and Accessories (4)**
   A. Beam Restriction
      1. light field to radiation field alignment
      2. central ray alignment
   B. Recognition and Reporting of Malfunctions
   C. Digital Imaging Receptor Systems
      1. artifacts (e.g., non-uniformity, erasure)
      2. maintenance (e.g., detector fog)
      3. display monitor quality assurance
   D. Shielding Accessories (e.g., lead apron and glove testing)

D. PATIENT CARE AND EDUCATION (17)

1. **Ethical and Legal Aspects (3)**
   A. Patient's Rights
      1. informed consent (e.g., written, oral, implied)
      2. confidentiality (HIPAA)
      3. additional rights (e.g., Patient's Bill of Rights)
         a. privacy
         b. extent of care (e.g., DNR)
         c. access to information
         d. living will; health care proxy
         e. research participation
   B. Legal Issues
      1. examination documentation (e.g., patient history, clinical diagnosis)
      2. common terminology (e.g., battery, negligence, malpractice)
      3. legal doctrines (e.g., *respondeat superior, res ipsa loquitur*)
      4. restraints versus immobilization
   C. Professional Ethics

2. **Interpersonal Communication (3)**
   A. Modes of Communication
      1. verbal/written
      2. nonverbal (e.g., eye contact, touching)
   B. Challenges in Communication
      1. patient characteristics
      2. explanation of medical terms
      3. strategies to improve understanding
      4. cultural diversity
   C. Patient Education (e.g., explanation of current procedure)

3. **Infection Control (5)**
   A. Terminology and Basic Concepts
      1. asepsis
         a. medical
         b. surgical
         c. sterile technique
      2. pathogens
         a. fomites, vehicles, vectors
         b. nosocomial infections
   B. Cycle of Infection
      1. pathogen
      2. source or reservoir of infection
      3. susceptible host
      4. method of transmission
         a. contact (direct, indirect)
         b. droplet
         c. airborne/suspended
         d. common vehicle
         e. vector borne
   C. Standard Precautions
      1. handwashing
      2. gloves, gowns
      3. masks
      4. medical asepsis (e.g., equipment disinfection)
   D. Additional or Transmission-Based Precautions
      1. airborne (e.g., respiratory protection, negative ventilation)
      2. droplet (e.g., mask, restricted patient placement)
      3. contact (e.g., gloves, gown, restricted patient placement)
   E. Disposal of Contaminated Materials
      1. linens
      2. needles
      3. patient supplies (e.g., tubes, emesis basin)

4. **Physical Assistance and Transfer (3)**
   A. Patient Transfer and Movement
      1. body mechanics (balance, alignment, movement)
      2. patient transfer
   B. Assisting Patients with Medical Equipment (e.g., oxygen delivery systems)
   C. Routine Monitoring
      1. equipment (e.g., stethoscope, sphygmomanometer)
      2. vital signs (e.g., blood pressure, pulse, respiration)
      3. physical signs and symptoms (e.g., motor control, severity of injury)
      4. documentation

5. **Medical Emergencies (3)**
   A. Allergic Reactions (e.g., latex)
   B. Cardiac or Respiratory Arrest (e.g., CPR)
   C. Physical Injury or Trauma
   D. Other Medical Disorders (e.g., seizures, diabetic reactions)

E. SPECIFIC IMAGING PROCEDURES

The specific positions and projections within each anatomic region that may be covered on the examination are listed in Attachment A. A guide to positioning terminology appears in Attachment B.

Radiographic Procedure Module[1]	# Questions Per Module[2]		Focus of Questions[3]
1. **Chest**			1. **Positioning** (topographic landmarks, body positions, path of central ray, etc.)
A. Routine	16		
B. Other	4		
TOTAL	20		emphasis: high
2. **Extremities**			
A. Lower (toes, foot, calcaneus, ankle, tibia, fibula, knee, patella, and distal femur)	11		2. **Anatomy** (including physiology, basic pathology, and related medical terminology)
B. Upper (fingers, hand, wrist, forearm, elbow, and humerus)	11		
C. Pectoral Girdle (shoulder, scapula, clavicle, and acromioclavicular joints)	3		emphasis: medium
TOTAL	25		
3. **Skull/Sinuses**	8		3. **Technical Factors** (including adjustments for circumstances such as body habitus, trauma, pathology, breathing techniques, casts, splints, soft tissue for foreign body, etc.)
A. Skull	8		
B. Paranasal Sinuses			
C. Facial Bones (nasal bones, orbits)	4		
TOTAL	20		
4. **Spine**	8		emphasis: low
A. Cervical Spine	6		
B. Thoracic Spine	8		
C. Lumbar Spine			4. **Equipment and Accessories** (grids or Bucky, compensating filter, automatic exposure control [AEC], automatic collimation, dedicated chest unit)
D. Sacrum, Coccyx, and Sacroiliac Joints	2		
E. Scoliosis Series	1		
TOTAL	25		
5. **Podiatric**	14		
A. Foot and Toes	5		
B. Ankle	1		emphasis: low
C. Calcaneus (os calcis)			
TOTAL	20		

Notes:

1. Examinees take one or more anatomic modules, depending on the type of license they have applied for. Each radiographic procedure module has 20 or 25 scored test questions, depending on the module (see chart above). The number of questions <u>within</u> a module should be regarded as approximate values.

2. Each of the radiographic procedure modules has five additional unscored questions.

3. The anatomic modules may include questions about the four areas listed under *FOCUS OF QUESTIONS* on the right side of the chart. The podiatric module does <u>not</u> include questions from the equipment and accessories section.

ARRT Content Specifications for the Limited Scope of Practice in Radiography Examination

I. **Chest**
A. Chest
1. PA or AP upright
2. lateral upright
3. AP lordotic
4. AP supine
5. lateral decubitus
6. anterior and posterior oblique

II. **Extremities**
A. Toes
1. AP, entire foot
2. oblique toe
3. lateral toe

B. Foot
1. AP angle toward heel
2. medial oblique
3. lateral oblique
4. mediolateral
5. lateromedial
6. sesamoids, tangential
7. AP weight bearing
8. lateral weight bearing

C. Calcaneus (Os Calcis)
1. lateral
2. plantodorsal, axial
3. dorsoplantar, axial

D. Ankle
1. AP
2. AP oblique mortise
3. mediolateral
4. oblique, 45° internal (medial)
5. lateromedial
6. AP stress views

E. Tibia, Fibula
1. AP
2. lateral
3. oblique

F. Knee
1. AP
2. lateral
3. AP weight bearing
4. lateral oblique 45°
5. medial oblique 45°
6. PA
7. PA axial—intercondylar fossa (tunnel)

G. Patella
1. lateral
2. supine flexion 45° (Merchant)
3. PA
4. prone flexion 90° (Settegast)
5. prone flexion 55° (Hughston)

H. Femur (Distal)
1. AP
2. mediolateral

I. Fingers
1. PA entire hand
2. PA finger only
3. lateral
4. oblique
5. AP thumb
6. oblique thumb
7. lateral thumb

J. Hand
1. PA
2. lateral
3. oblique

K. Wrist
1. PA
2. oblique 45°
3. lateral
4. PA for scaphoid
5. scaphoid (Stecher)
6. carpal canal

L. Forearm
1. AP
2. lateral

M. Elbow
1. AP
2. lateral
3. external (lateral) oblique
4. internal (medial) oblique
5. AP partial flexion
6. axial trauma (Coyle)

N. Humerus
1. AP
2. lateral
3. AP neutral
4. scapular Y
5. transthoracic lateral

O. Shoulder
1. AP internal and external rotation
2. inferosuperior axial
3. posterior oblique (Grashey)
4. tangential
5. AP neutral
6. transthoracic lateral
7. scapular Y

P. Scapula
1. AP
2. lateral, anterior oblique
3. lateral, posterior oblique

Q. Clavicle
1. AP
2. AP angle 15-30° cephalad
3. PA angle 15-30° caudad

R. Acromioclavicular joints
1. AP bilateral with and without weights

III. **Skull/Sinuses**
A. Skull
1. AP axial (Towne)
2. lateral
3. PA (Caldwell)
4. PA
5. submentovertical (full basal)

B. Facial Bones
1. lateral
2. parietoacanthial (Waters)
3. PA (Caldwell)
4. PA (modified Waters)

C. Nasal Bones
1. parietoacanthial (Waters)
2. lateral
3. PA (Caldwell)

D. Orbits
1. parietoacanthial (Waters)
2. lateral
3. PA (Caldwell)

E. Paranasal Sinuses
1. lateral
2. PA (Caldwell)
3. parietoacanthial (Waters)
4. submentovertical (full basal)
5. open mouth parietoacanthial (Waters)

IV. **Spine**
  A. Cervical cpine
    1. AP angle cephalad
    2. AP open mouth
    3. lateral
    4. anterior oblique
    5. posterior oblique
    6. lateral swimmers
    7. lateral flexion and extension
  B. Thoracic Spine
    1. AP
    2. lateral, breathing
    3. lateral, expiration
  C. Lumbar Spine
    1. AP
    2. PA
    3. lateral
    4. L5-S1 lateral spot
    5. posterior oblique 45°
    6. anterior oblique 45°
    7. AP L5-S1, 30-35° cephalad
    8. AP right and left bending
    9. lateral flexion and extension

  D. Sacrum and Coccyx
    1. AP sacrum, 15-25° cephalad
    2. AP coccyx, 10-20° caudad
    3. lateral sacrum and coccyx, combined
    4. lateral sacrum or coccyx, separate
  E. Sacroiliac Joints
    1. AP
    2. posterior oblique
    3. anterior oblique
  F. Scoliosis Series
    1. AP/PA scoliosis series (Ferguson)

V. **Podiatric**
  A. Foot and Toes
    1. dorsal plantar (DP)*
    2. medial oblique
    3. lateral oblique
    4. lateral
    5. sesamoidal axial*
  B. Ankle*
    1. AP*
    2. mortise*
    3. AP medial oblique*
    4. AP lateral oblique*
    5. lateral*
  C. Calcaneus (Os Calcis)
    1. axial calcaneal
    2. Harris and Beath (ski-jump)

---

* Weight bearing

ARRT Content Specifications for the Limited Scope of Practice in Radiography Examination

Attachment C
ARRT Standard Definitions

Term	Film-Screen Radiography	Term	Digital Radiography
Recorded Detail	The sharpness of the structural lines as recorded in the radiographic image.	Spatial Resolution	The sharpness of the structural edges recorded in the image.
Receptor Exposure	The amount of radiation striking the image receptor.	Receptor Exposure	The amount of radiation striking the image receptor.
Density	Radiographic density is the degree of blackening or opacity of an area in a radiograph due to the accumulation of black metallic silver following exposure and processing of a film. $$\text{Density} = \text{Log} \, \frac{\text{incident light intensity}}{\text{transmitted light intensity}}$$	Brightness	Brightness is the measurement of the luminance of a monitor calibrated in units of candela (cd) per square meter on a monitor or soft copy. Density on a hard copy is the same as film.
Contrast	Radiographic contrast is defined as the visible differences between any two selected areas of density levels within the radiographic image. Scale of Contrast refers to the number of densities visible (or the number of shades of gray). Long Scale is the term used when slight differences between densities are present (low contrast) but the total number of densities is increased. Short Scale is the term used when considerable or major differences between densities are present (high contrast) but the total number of densities is reduced.	Contrast	Image contrast or display contrast is determined primarily by the processing algorithm (mathematical codes used by the software to provide the desired image appearance). The default algorithm determines the initial processing codes applied to the image data. Scale of Contrast is synonymous to "gray scale" and is linked to the bit depth of the system. "Gray scale" is used instead of "scale of contrast" when referring to digital images.
Film Latitude	The inherent ability of the film to record a long range of density levels on the radiograph. Film latitude and film contrast depend upon the sensitometric properties of the film and the processing conditions and are determined directly from the characteristic H and D curve.	Dynamic Range	The range of exposures that may be captured by a detector. The dynamic range for digital imaging is much larger than film.
Film Contrast	The inherent ability of the film emulsion to react to radiation and record a range of densities.	Receptor Contrast	The fixed characteristic of the receptor. Most digital receptors have an essentially linear response to exposure. This is impacted by **contrast resolution** (the smallest exposure change or signal difference that can be detected). Ultimately, contrast resolution is limited by the dynamic range and the **quantization** (number of bits per pixel) of the detector.
Exposure Latitude	The range of exposure factors which will produce a diagnostic radiograph.	Exposure Latitude	The range of exposures which produces quality images at appropriate patient dose.
Subject Contrast	The difference in the quantity of radiation transmitted by a particular part as a result of the different absorption characteristics of the tissues and structures making up that part.	Subject Contrast	The magnitude of the signal difference in the remnant beam.

Simulated Examination for the Limited Scope of Practice in Radiography

Complete this examination in pencil if you plan to take it more than once. If you are not sure of the answer to a question, skip it and return to it after completing the entire examination.

Multiple Choice

Identify the choice that best completes the statement or answers the question.

_____ 1. Which of the following statements are correct regarding the link between radiation dose and genetic effects?
1. The link has been demonstrated in human studies.
2. The link has been demonstrated in animal studies.
3. Increased risk to humans cannot be predicted with respect to an individual.
A. 1 and 2 only
B. 1 and 3 only
C. 2 and 3 only
D. 1, 2, and 3

_____ 2. Which of the following changes in kilovoltage (kVp) will result in the greatest reduction of patient dose, when milliampere-seconds (mAs) is adjusted to compensate for the change?
A. Decrease kVp by 30%.
B. Decrease kVp by 15%.
C. Increase kVp by 15%.
D. Increase kVp by 30%.

_____ 3. Which of the following image receptor (IR) system speeds will result in the lowest patient dose?
A. Slower-speed IR system
B. Faster-speed IR system
C. It does not matter; the IR system speed does not affect the patient dose.

_____ 4. What is the primary purpose of using gonad shields during radiography?
A. Reduce the likelihood of genetic effects
B. Reduce the likelihood of somatic effects
C. Protect patient modesty
D. Demonstrate the location of the gonads in the image

_____ 5. Which of the following are types of gonad shields?
1. Aperture
2. Contact
3. Shadow
A. 1 and 2 only
B. 1 and 3 only
C. 2 and 3 only
D. 1, 2, and 3

_____ 6. When should gonad shielding be used?
A. For all patients
B. For all procedures
C. When the gonads are within 10 cm of the radiation field
D. When the gonads are within 5 cm of the radiation field

_____ 7. The greatest cause of unnecessary radiation to patients that can be controlled by the limited operator is:
A. patient condition.
B. patient size.
C. repeat exposures.
D. equipment malfunction.

_____ 8. The limited operator can reduce repeat exposures by:
A. accepting marginal images.
B. clearly instructing patients.
C. increasing the source–image receptor distance (SID).
D. optimizing the kVp.

_____ 9. How does x-ray beam restriction minimize patient exposure?
A. It limits radiation fog.
B. It limits the radiation field to the area of interest.
C. It limits the effect of patient motion.
D. It limits repeat exposures.

_____ 10. What is the device that allows the limited operator to vary the size of the radiation field?
A. Collimator
B. Detent
C. Filter
D. Shield

255

11. How does filtration reduce patient exposure?
    A. Removes shorter-wavelength photons
    B. Removes longer-wavelength photons
    C. Reduces the size of the radiation field
    D. Reduces the time of exposure

12. What is the National Council on Radiation Protection and Measurements (NCRP) recommendation for the amount of total filtration?
    A. 0.5 mm aluminum equivalent (Al equiv)
    B. 1.5 mm Al equiv
    C. 2.5 mm Al equiv
    D. 3.5 mm Al equiv

13. What are the three principal methods used to protect limited operators from unnecessary radiation exposure?
    A. Time, distance, and shielding
    B. Time, distance, and collimation
    C. Distance, collimation, and shielding
    D. Time, collimation, and filtration

14. Which of the following is *not* a type of personnel radiation shielding?
    A. Apron
    B. Glove
    C. Thyroid shield
    D. Shadow

15. Personnel shielding must be worn on the rare occasion during which the limited operator may need to remain in the radiographic room during an exposure to assist the patient in maintaining the proper position. What is the source of the greatest radiation hazard under this circumstance?
    A. Off-focus radiation
    B. Leakage radiation
    C. Scattered radiation from the patient
    D. Backscatter radiation from the IR

16. What is the term for radiation that escapes from the x-ray tube housing?
    A. Scattered radiation
    B. Off-focus radiation
    C. Primary radiation
    D. Leakage radiation

17. Why are limited operators prohibited from activities that result in direct exposure to the primary x-ray beam?
    A. They are considered occupationally exposed individuals.
    B. These activities carry immediate health risks.
    C. Their interaction with the beam will affect patient dose.
    D. Their presence near the patient increases liability.

18. Distance, as a method used to limit operator exposure, means that:
    A. the operator should maximize the distance from the source during an exposure.
    B. the operator should minimize the distance from the source during an exposure.
    C. the operator should maximize the distance from the patient during an exposure.
    D. the operator should minimize the distance from the patient during an exposure.

19. Shielding worn for personnel protection is designed to attenuate what source of exposure?
    A. Primary radiation
    B. Off-focus radiation
    C. Leakage radiation
    D. Scatter radiation

20. Which of the following is an acronym for a common type of personnel dosimeter?
    A. TLC
    B. TLD
    C. OSD
    D. OID

21. What is the recommended placement for a personnel dosimeter on the body of the limited operator?
    A. The badge should be worn in the region of the waist on the anterior surface of the body and outside the lead apron, if worn.
    B. The badge should be worn in the region of the waist on the posterior surface of the body and inside the lead apron, if worn.
    C. The badge should be worn in the region of the collar on the posterior surface of the body and inside the lead apron, if worn.
    D. The badge should be worn in the region of the collar on the anterior surface of the body and outside the lead apron, if worn.

22. What is the NCRP recommended annual effective dose limit for occupational exposure?
    A. 0.05 roentgen equivalent man (rem) (0.0005 sievert [Sv])
    B. 0.5 rem (0.005 Sv)
    C. 5.0 rem (0.05 Sv)
    D. 50.0 rem (0.5 Sv)

23. What is the NCRP recommended monthly effective (or equivalent) dose limit to the fetus for a pregnant worker?
    A. 0.05 rem (0.0005 Sv)
    B. 0.5 rem (0.005 Sv)
    C. 5.0 rem (0.05 Sv)
    D. 50.0 rem (0.5 Sv)

24. Radiation monitoring of personnel is required when what percentage of the annual occupational effective dose limit is likely to be received?
   A. 5%
   B. 10%
   C. 15%
   D. 20%

25. What is the conventional (British system) radiation unit to express radiation intensity in air?
   A. Coulomb/kilogram (C/kg)
   B. Watt
   C. Ohm
   D. Roentgen

26. The conventional (British system) unit commonly used to report occupational dose to radiation workers in the United States is the:
   A. mR.
   B. rad.
   C. rem.
   D. mGy.

27. What is the conventional (British system) radiation unit of absorbed dose?
   A. Rad
   B. Roentgen
   C. Gray
   D. Rem

28. According to the Bergonié–Tribondeau law, which of the following types of cells are most radiosensitive?
   A. Brain cells
   B. Embryonic tissue cells
   C. Cells of the gastric mucosa
   D. Skin cells

29. Which type of x-ray photon interaction with the body is primarily responsible for the radiation dose absorbed by the patient?
   A. Compton
   B. Photoelectric
   C. Coherent
   D. Characteristic

30. What is the NCRP (report #102) recommendation for lead equivalency of aprons used for personnel protection?
   A. 0.05 mm
   B. 0.25 mm
   C. 0.5 mm
   D. 1.0 mm

31. What is erythema, as it relates to radiation exposure?
   A. Loss of hair caused by a high radiation dose
   B. Loss of hair caused by a long-term low radiation dose
   C. Reddening of the skin caused by a high radiation dose
   D. Reddening of the skin caused by a long-term low radiation dose

32. What is the guiding philosophy of radiation protection?
   A. ALARMA—as long as radiographs are made accessible
   B. ALARA—as low as reasonably achievable
   C. ALAIS—as long as ionizations are small
   D. ALAP—as low as possible

33. Which of the following statements reflects current scientific opinion regarding the effects of diagnostic levels of ionizing radiation?
   A. It is carcinogenic after a certain number of examinations have been performed.
   B. Spontaneous abortion will occur if the patient is pregnant.
   C. Depression of the white blood cell count is followed by acute gastrointestinal distress.
   D. There is an increased risk of cancer, leukemia, birth defects, and cataracts.

34. Which of the following changes will decrease patient dose?
   1. Using a faster-speed class imaging system
   2. Increasing the kVp using the 15% rule, while decreasing the mAs to compensate
   3. Increasing the grid ratio to a 16:1 ratio
   A. 1 and 2 only
   B. 1 and 3 only
   C. 2 and 3 only
   D. 1, 2, and 3

35. When radiation exposure occurs during pregnancy, the greatest risk of birth defects occurs when the exposure:
   1. exceeds 5 rad to the uterus.
   2. occurs within the first trimester of pregnancy.
   3. occurs within the third trimester of pregnancy.
   A. 1 and 2 only
   B. 1 and 3 only
   C. 2 and 3 only
   D. 1, 2, and 3

66. What conditions are most important for optimum viewing of radiographic images?
    A. Low room temperature
    B. High room humidity
    C. Low room light level
    D. Bright room light level

67. Marks, exposures, or images on a radiograph that are not a part of the intended image are called:
    A. fog.
    B. ghosts.
    C. phantoms.
    D. artifacts.

68. If the amount of irradiated tissue increases, what happens to scatter radiation fog?
    A. There is not enough information provided to answer the question.
    B. Scatter radiation fog increases.
    C. Scatter radiation fog decreases.
    D. Scatter radiation fog is not affected by the amount of tissue irradiated.

69. The most effective and practical way to reduce scatter radiation fog on a radiograph is to:
    A. decrease the OID.
    B. decrease the SID.
    C. increase the kVp.
    D. use a grid or Bucky.

70. As a general rule, a grid should be employed when the part thickness is greater than:
    A. 4 cm.
    B. 12 cm.
    C. 18 cm.
    D. 12 inches.

71. Technique charts are based on patient part measurements obtained using an x-ray caliper and are expressed as:
    A. circumference in inches.
    B. thickness in centimeters.
    C. diameter in millimeters.
    D. depth in inches.

72. Which of the following pathologic conditions would require a decrease in exposure?
    1. Multiple myeloma
    2. Emphysema
    3. Osteoporosis
    A. 1 and 2 only
    B. 1 and 3 only
    C. 2 and 3 only
    D. 1, 2, and 3

73. How will the anode heel effect, if present, be seen on an image?
    A. The image will have higher contrast on the anode end than on the cathode end.
    B. The image will have lower contrast on the anode end than on the cathode end.
    C. The image will be darker on the anode end than on the cathode end.
    D. The image will be lighter on the anode end than on the cathode end.

74. Which radiographic quality factor is most affected by angulation of the central ray, part, or IR?
    A. Receptor exposure
    B. Contrast
    C. Spatial resolution
    D. Distortion

75. What is the recommendation for a hard-copy image that is mislabeled?
    A. The image must be repeated to ensure a correct, permanent label.
    B. A sticker with the correct information should be applied to the hard copy image.
    C. The correct information should be handwritten on the hard copy image.
    D. No correction is needed.

76. Which of the following will result in a screen or film image with low density?
    A. IR exposure with collimation wider than needed for the particular anatomic structures
    B. IR exposure with a kVp higher than needed for the particular anatomic structures
    C. IR exposure at an SID closer than expected for the exposure factors selected
    D. IR exposure with an mAs less than needed for the particular anatomic structures

77. Which of the following will result in a screen or film image with low contrast?
    A. IR exposure with collimation smaller than needed for the particular anatomic structures
    B. IR exposure with mAs higher than needed for the particular anatomic structures
    C. IR exposure at an SID closer than expected for the exposure factors selected
    D. IR exposure with a kVp higher than needed for the particular anatomic structures

78. When viewing a digital image on a monitor, how do you determine if the proper mAs was selected?
   A. Evaluate the image brightness.
   B. Evaluate the image contrast.
   C. Evaluate the image distortion.
   D. Evaluate the exposure index value.

79. Which of the following will result in an image with poor spatial resolution?
   A. IR exposure with collimation wider than needed for the particular anatomic structures
   B. IR exposure with mAs higher than needed for the particular anatomic structures
   C. IR exposure with a kVp higher than needed for the particular anatomic structures
   D. Patient motion

80. Which of the following will result in an image with excessive magnification of image structures?
   A. IR exposure with a kVp higher than needed for the particular anatomic structures
   B. IR exposure at an SID greater than recommended for a particular body part
   C. IR exposure at an OID greater than recommended for a particular body part
   D. IR exposure with mAs higher than needed for the particular anatomic structures

81. Which of the following will result in an image with excessive distortion of anatomic structures?
   A. Improper central ray angulation for the selected radiographic projection
   B. Use of an 8:1 grid with the mAs set for a 12:1 grid
   C. IR exposure at an SID greater than recommended for a particular body part
   D. IR exposure with the mAs higher than needed for the particular anatomic structures

82. Poor film or screen contact is seen on a radiograph as a decrease in what radiographic quality factor?
   A. Density or brightness
   B. Contrast or gray scale
   C. Recorded detail or spatial resolution
   D. Distortion

83. Which screen film image artifact looks like lightning?
   A. Static artifact
   B. Handling artifact
   C. Pressure artifact
   D. Chemical artifact

84. Which of the following would be a violation of patient confidentiality?
   A. A limited operator discusses a patient's existing pathology with a radiographer to get assistance in setting technical factors.
   B. A limited operator talks to his or her friend during lunch about a patient's imaging procedure.
   C. A radiographer asks if a patient is pregnant before an acute abdominal series.
   D. A transporter tells the limited operator that the patient complained of dizziness while riding in the wheelchair to the x-ray department.

85. Which of the following are true regarding informed consent?
   1. Informed consent may be revoked at any time.
   2. The patient must be legally competent to sign.
   3. The patient may sign an incomplete form and the blanks may be filled in later by the physician.
   A. 1 and 2 only
   B. 1 and 3 only
   C. 2 and 3 only
   D. 1, 2, and 3

86. A limited operator innocently commits an error as a result of following the orders of his or her employer, a physician. The employer may be held responsible according to the:
   A. American Society of Radiologic Technologists code of ethics.
   B. rule of professional responsibility.
   C. doctrine of respondeat superior.
   D. doctrine of *non compos mentis.*

87. Communication has been "validated" when the speaker has:
   A. spoken clearly.
   B. received a response from the listener that demonstrates comprehension.
   C. presented the information accurately.
   D. reviewed the material.

88. Which of the following is *not* a form of nonverbal communication?
   A. Speaking
   B. Touching
   C. Eye contact
   D. Facial expression

89. Mrs. Elizabeth Dunbar is 86 years old and a bit confused. She is most likely to respond appropriately if you address her as:
    A. Betty.
    B. Honey.
    C. Mrs. Dunbar.
    D. Elizabeth.

90. Which of the following are correct statements of proper body mechanics?
    1. Use a broad stance.
    2. Turn and lift using your back muscles.
    3. Carry heavy objects close to your body.
    A. 1 and 2 only
    B. 1 and 3 only
    C. 2 and 3 only
    D. 1, 2, and 3

91. What type of disease transmission is possible when the limited operator does not clean the Bucky device after performing an examination on a patient with influenza?
    A. Vector transmission
    B. Direct contact transmission
    C. Indirect contact or fomite transmission
    D. Airborne transmission

92. Standard precautions involve the use of barriers whenever contact is anticipated with:
    1. blood.
    2. body fluids.
    3. mucous membranes.
    A. 1 and 2 only
    B. 1 and 3 only
    C. 2 and 3 only
    D. 1, 2, and 3

93. The process of reducing the probability that infectious organisms will be transmitted to a susceptible individual is called:
    A. sepsis.
    B. asepsis.
    C. inoculation.
    D. vaccination.

94. A health care worker's single best protection against disease is:
    A. frequent hand washing.
    B. vaccination.
    C. barrier techniques.
    D. protective masks.

95. A limited operator who does not change linens between patients is:
    A. providing an opportunity for fomite transmission.
    B. saving money on laundry expenses.
    C. making wise decisions, as long as there are no stains on the linens.
    D. increasing productivity by saving time between patients.

96. What is anaphylaxis?
    A. The absence of a pain response
    B. A severe allergic reaction
    C. Complete unconsciousness
    D. Inability to breathe

97. What is the basic life support system used to ventilate the lungs and circulate the blood in the event of cardiac or respiratory arrest?
    A. Cardiac tamponade
    B. AED
    C. CPR
    D. ACLS

98. When a patient in cardiac arrest presents with a rapid, weak, and ineffective heartbeat, what device is used to return the heart to a normal rhythm?
    A. Cardiac tamponade
    B. AED
    C. CPR
    D. ACLS

99. Which of the following vital signs can be assessed without touching the patient?
    A. Pulse
    B. Respiration
    C. Blood pressure
    D. Temperature

100. What is the most common site for palpation of a patient's pulse?
    A. Carotid artery
    B. Apex of the heart
    C. Dorsalis pedis
    D. Radial artery at the wrist

Simulated Examination for the Limited Scope of Practice in Radiography—Core Module

Answer Section

Multiple Choice

1. **ANS: C**	REF: Ch. 11	OBJ: exam spec A.1.E.1	TOP: radiation biology
2. **ANS: D**	REF: Ch. 11	OBJ: exam spec A.2.A.1	TOP: patient exposure
3. **ANS: B**	REF: Ch. 11	OBJ: exam spec A.2.F	TOP: patient exposure
4. **ANS: A**	REF: Ch. 11	OBJ: exam spec A.2.B.1	TOP: patient exposure
5. **ANS: C**	REF: Ch. 11	OBJ: exam spec A.2.B.2	TOP: patient exposure
6. **ANS: D**	REF: Ch. 11	OBJ: exam spec A.2.B.3	TOP: patient exposure
7. **ANS: C**	REF: Ch. 11	OBJ: exam spec A.2.E.5	TOP: patient exposure
8. **ANS: B**	REF: Ch. 11	OBJ: exam spec A.2.E.2	TOP: patient exposure
9. **ANS: B**	REF: Ch. 11	OBJ: exam spec A.2.C.1	TOP: patient exposure
10. **ANS: A**	REF: Ch. 2	OBJ: exam spec A.2.C.2	TOP: patient exposure
11. **ANS: B**	REF: Ch. 5	OBJ: exam spec A.2.D.2	TOP: patient exposure
12. **ANS: C**	REF: Ch. 5	OBJ: exam spec A.2.D.3	TOP: patient exposure
13. **ANS: A**	REF: Ch. 11	OBJ: exam spec A.3.B	TOP: personnel protection
14. **ANS: D**	REF: Ch. 11	OBJ: exam spec A.3.B.3	TOP: personnel protection
15. **ANS: C**	REF: Ch. 11	OBJ: exam spec A.3.B.3	TOP: personnel protection
16. **ANS: D**	REF: Ch. 11	OBJ: exam spec A.3.A.2.b	TOP: personnel protection
17. **ANS: A**	REF: Ch. 11	OBJ: exam spec A.3.A.1	TOP: personnel protection
18. **ANS: A**	REF: Ch. 11	OBJ: exam spec A.3.B.2	TOP: personnel protection
19. **ANS: D**	REF: Ch. 11	OBJ: exam spec A.3.B.3	TOP: personnel protection
20. **ANS: B**	REF: Ch. 11	OBJ: exam spec A.4.B.1	TOP: radiation exposure/monitoring
21. **ANS: D**	REF: Ch. 11	OBJ: exam spec A.4.B.2	TOP: radiation exposure/monitoring
22. **ANS: C**	REF: Ch. 11	OBJ: exam spec A.4.C.1	TOP: radiation exposure/monitoring
23. **ANS: A**	REF: Ch. 11	OBJ: exam spec A.4.C.3	TOP: radiation exposure/monitoring
24. **ANS: B**	REF: Ch. 11	OBJ: exam spec A.4.C.4	TOP: radiation exposure/monitoring
25. **ANS: D**	REF: Ch. 11	OBJ: exam spec A.4.A.3	TOP: radiation exposure/monitoring
26. **ANS: C**	REF: Ch. 11	OBJ: exam spec A.4.A.2	TOP: radiation exposure/monitoring
27. **ANS: A**	REF: Ch. 11	OBJ: exam spec A.4.A.1	TOP: radiation exposure/monitoring
28. **ANS: B**	REF: Ch. 11	OBJ: exam spec A.1.A.2	TOP: radiation biology
29. **ANS: B**	REF: Ch. 11	OBJ: exam spec A.1.F.2	TOP: radiation biology
30. **ANS: C**	REF: Ch. 11	OBJ: exam spec A.3.C.3	TOP: personnel protection
31. **ANS: C**	REF: Ch. 11	OBJ: exam spec A.1.B.2	TOP: radiation biology
32. **ANS: B**	REF: Ch. 11	OBJ: exam spec A.2.E.5	TOP: patient exposure
33. **ANS: D**	REF: Ch. 11	OBJ: exam spec A.1.B.3	TOP: radiation biology
34. **ANS: A**	REF: Ch. 11	OBJ: exam spec A.2.F	TOP: patient exposure
35. **ANS: A**	REF: Ch. 11	OBJ: exam spec A.1.D	TOP: radiation biology
36. **ANS: D**	REF: Ch. 9	OBJ: exam spec A.1.F.1	TOP: radiation biology
37. **ANS: B**	REF: Ch. 9	OBJ: exam spec A.3.A.3	TOP: personnel protection
38. **ANS: A**	REF: Ch. 5	OBJ: exam spec B.1.A	TOP: radiation physics
39. **ANS: B**	REF: Ch. 5	OBJ: exam spec B.1.B	TOP: radiation physics
40. **ANS: D**	REF: Ch. 5	OBJ: exam spec B.1.C.2.a	TOP: radiation physics
41. **ANS: A**	REF: Ch. 6	OBJ: exam spec B.2.B	TOP: imaging equipment
42. **ANS: D**	REF: Ch. 6	OBJ: exam spec B.2.C.1	TOP: imaging equipment
43. **ANS: D**	REF: Ch. 6	OBJ: exam spec B.2.B	TOP: imaging equipment
44. **ANS: A**	REF: Ch. 6	OBJ: exam spec B.2.A.2.b	TOP: imaging equipment
45. **ANS: C**	REF: Ch. 9	OBJ: exam spec B.3.A.1	TOP: equipment quality control
46. **ANS: B**	REF: Ch. 9	OBJ: exam spec B.3.A.2	TOP: equipment quality control
47. **ANS: B**	REF: Ch. 11	OBJ: exam spec B.3.D	TOP: equipment quality control
48. **ANS: C**	REF: Ch. 8	OBJ: exam spec B.3.C.2	TOP: equipment quality control
49. **ANS: D**	REF: Ch. 7	OBJ: exam spec C.1.A.a	TOP: technical factor selection
50. **ANS: D**	REF: Ch. 7	OBJ: exam spec C.1.A.a	TOP: technical factor selection
51. **ANS: B**	REF: Ch. 7	OBJ: exam spec C.1.A.d	TOP: technical factor selection
52. **ANS: C**	REF: Ch. 7	OBJ: exam spec C.1.A	TOP: technical factor selection
53. **ANS: C**	REF: Ch. 7	OBJ: exam spec C.1.A.b	TOP: technical factor selection

12. What is the purpose of rotating the patient's shoulders anteriorly for the PA projection of the chest?
    A. This motion rotates the scapulae out of the lungs.
    B. This motion reduces magnification of the heart shadow.
    C. This motion makes the position more comfortable for the patient.
    D. This motion places the coronal plane parallel to the upright grid cabinet.

13. Where does the central ray enter the patient for the upright, PA projection of the chest?
    A. Midsagittal plane at the level of T7
    B. Midcoronal plane at the level of T7
    C. Midsagittal plane at the level of the iliac crests
    D. Midcoronal plane at the level of the iliac crests

14. What is the proper placement of the arms for the upright lateral projection of the chest?
    A. Backs of the hands on the hips with the shoulders rolled anteriorly
    B. Arms raised over the head with the hands grasping opposite elbows
    C. Arms abducted from the thorax
    D. Arms adducted from the thorax

15. What are the proper patient instructions for the PA projection of the chest?
    A. Stop breathing after the second deep inspiration.
    B. Stop breathing after deep inspiration.
    C. Stop breathing after expiration.
    D. Breathe slowly and evenly.

16. Lateral projections of the chest are taken with the left side against the IR because:
    A. lung pathology is more common on the left side.
    B. it is conventional to have a routine standard, and the left has been established as the standard.
    C. magnification of the cardiac silhouette is reduced with the left side nearer the IR.
    D. the right hilum provides high-contrast details that may be confusing.

17. How much should the central ray be angled cephalad for an AP axial projection of the chest if the patient cannot assume the lordotic position?
    A. No angle is needed
    B. 10 degrees
    C. 15 degrees
    D. 25 degrees

18. Which chest projection and position are needed to demonstrate free pleural fluid along the dependent chest wall?
    A. AP, upright
    B. PA, recumbent
    C. AP, lordotic
    D. AP, lateral decubitus

19. Which of the following projections is best for demonstration of the apices of the lungs without bony superimposition?
    A. PA
    B. Lateral
    C. AP axial, lordotic position
    D. PA oblique

20. Why is a grid used for routine chest radiography?
    A. To reduce scatter fog caused by use of a high kVp
    B. To reduce the patient dose by filtration
    C. To reduce magnification caused by an increased SID
    D. To increase the recorded detail

Answer Section

Multiple Choice

1. **ANS: C**	REF: Ch. 12	OBJ: exam spec E.1.A.1	TOP: routine chest positioning
2. **ANS: D**	REF: Ch. 16	OBJ: exam spec E.1.A.2	TOP: chest anatomy
3. **ANS: C**	REF: Ch. 16	OBJ: exam spec E.1.A.2	TOP: chest anatomy
4. **ANS: A**	REF: Ch. 16	OBJ: exam spec E.1.A.2	TOP: chest anatomy
5. **ANS: C**	REF: Ch. 16	OBJ: exam spec E.1.A.2	TOP: chest anatomy
6. **ANS: D**	REF: Ch. 16	OBJ: exam spec E.1.A.2	TOP: chest anatomy
7. **ANS: D**	REF: Ch. 16	OBJ: exam spec E.1.A.1	TOP: routine chest positioning
8. **ANS: C**	REF: Ch. 16	OBJ: exam spec E.1.A.1	TOP: routine chest positioning
9. **ANS: D**	REF: Ch. 16	OBJ: exam spec E.1.A.1	TOP: routine chest positioning
10. **ANS: D**	REF: Ch. 16	OBJ: exam spec E.1.A.1	TOP: routine chest positioning
11. **ANS: A**	REF: Ch. 16	OBJ: exam spec E.1.A.3	TOP: routine chest technical factors
12. **ANS: A**	REF: Ch. 16	OBJ: exam spec E.1.A.1	TOP: routine chest positioning
13. **ANS: A**	REF: Ch. 16	OBJ: exam spec E.1.A.1	TOP: routine chest positioning
14. **ANS: B**	REF: Ch. 16	OBJ: exam spec E.1.A.1	TOP: routine chest positioning
15. **ANS: A**	REF: Ch. 16	OBJ: exam spec E.1.A.1	TOP: routine chest positioning
16. **ANS: C**	REF: Ch. 16	OBJ: exam spec E.1.A.1	TOP: routine chest positioning
17. **ANS: C**	REF: Ch. 16	OBJ: exam spec E.1.B.1	TOP: other chest positioning
18. **ANS: D**	REF: Ch. 16	OBJ: exam spec E.1.B.1	TOP: other chest positioning
19. **ANS: C**	REF: Ch. 16	OBJ: exam spec E.1.B.1	TOP: other chest positioning
20. **ANS: A**	REF: Ch. 16	OBJ: exam spec E.1.A.4	TOP: routine chest equipment

SIMULATED EXAMINATION FOR THE LIMITED SCOPE OF PRACTICE IN RADIOGRAPHY— EXTREMITIES MODULE

Complete this examination in pencil if you plan to take it more than once. If you are not sure of the answer to a question, skip it and return to it after completing the entire examination.

Multiple Choice
Identify the choice that best completes the statement or answers the question.

_____ 1. Which of the following bones are in the hindfoot portion of the foot?
  1. Cuneiforms
  2. Calcaneus
  3. Talus
  A. 1 and 2 only
  B. 1 and 3 only
  C. 2 and 3 only
  D. 1, 2, and 3

_____ 2. The anatomic name for the bone commonly known as the *kneecap* is the:
  A. fibula.
  B. tibia.
  C. patella.
  D. fabella.

_____ 3. The palpable portion at the distal end of the tibia is called the:
  A. lateral malleolus.
  B. medial malleolus.
  C. medial condyle.
  D. lateral condyle.

_____ 4. When the ankle is flexed to raise the foot, the movement is termed:
  A. plantar flexion.
  B. eversion.
  C. inversion.
  D. dorsiflexion.

_____ 5. What device may help provide an even density on a radiograph of an anteroposterior (AP) axial projection of the foot?
  A. Lead shield
  B. Wedge compensating filter
  C. Wedge positioning sponge
  D. Sandbag

Answer Section

Multiple Choice

1. ANS: C	REF: Ch. 14	OBJ: exam spec E.2.A.2	TOP: lower extremity anatomy
2. ANS: C	REF: Ch. 14	OBJ: exam spec E.2.A.2	TOP: lower extremity anatomy
3. ANS: B	REF: Ch. 14	OBJ: exam spec E.2.A.2	TOP: lower extremity anatomy
4. ANS: D	REF: Ch. 14	OBJ: exam spec E.2.A.1	TOP: lower extremity positioning
5. ANS: B	REF: Ch. 14	OBJ: exam spec E.2.A.4	TOP: lower extremity accessory equipment
6. ANS: C	REF: Ch. 14	OBJ: exam spec E.2.A.1	TOP: lower extremity positioning
7. ANS: A	REF: Ch. 14	OBJ: exam spec E.2.A.1	TOP: lower extremity positioning
8. ANS: A	REF: Ch. 14	OBJ: exam spec E.2.A.1	TOP: lower extremity positioning
9. ANS: A	REF: Ch. 14	OBJ: exam spec E.2.A.1	TOP: lower extremity positioning
10. ANS: D	REF: Ch. 14	OBJ: exam spec E.2.A.1	TOP: lower extremity positioning
11. ANS: A	REF: Ch. 10	OBJ: exam spec E.2.A.3	TOP: lower extremity technical factors
12. ANS: C	REF: Ch. 13	OBJ: exam spec E.2.B.2	TOP: upper extremity anatomy
13. ANS: A	REF: Ch. 13	OBJ: exam spec E.2.B.2	TOP: upper extremity anatomy
14. ANS: D	REF: Ch. 13	OBJ: exam spec E.2.B.2	TOP: upper extremity anatomy
15. ANS: D	REF: Ch. 13	OBJ: exam spec E.2.B.1	TOP: upper extremity positioning
16. ANS: A	REF: Ch. 13	OBJ: exam spec E.2.B.1	TOP: upper extremity positioning
17. ANS: A	REF: Ch. 13	OBJ: exam spec E.2.B.1	TOP: upper extremity positioning
18. ANS: C	REF: Ch. 13	OBJ: exam spec E.2.B.1	TOP: upper extremity positioning
19. ANS: A	REF: Ch. 13	OBJ: exam spec E.2.B.1	TOP: upper extremity positioning
20. ANS: B	REF: Ch. 13	OBJ: exam spec E.2.B.1	TOP: upper extremity positioning
21. ANS: A	REF: Ch. 13	OBJ: exam spec E.2.B.1	TOP: upper extremity positioning
22. ANS: A	REF: Ch. 10	OBJ: exam spec E.2.B.3	TOP: upper extremity technical factors
23. ANS: B	REF: Ch. 13	OBJ: exam spec E.2.C.1	TOP: shoulder positioning
24. ANS: A	REF: Ch. 13	OBJ: exam spec E.2.C.1	TOP: shoulder positioning
25. ANS: C	REF: Ch. 13	OBJ: exam spec E.2.C.2	TOP: shoulder anatomy

SIMULATED EXAMINATION FOR THE LIMITED SCOPE OF PRACTICE IN RADIOGRAPHY—SKULL/SINUSES MODULE

Complete this examination in pencil if you plan to take it more than once. If you are not sure of the answer to a question, skip it and return to it after completing the entire examination.

Multiple Choice
Identify the choice that best completes the statement or answers the question.

_____ 1. Which of the following cranial bones are paired (right and left)?
1. Frontal
2. Parietal
3. Temporal
A. 1 only
B. 1 and 2 only
C. 2 and 3 only
D. 1, 2, and 3

_____ 2. What structure serves as the passageway for the spinal cord to exit the skull and pass into the spinal canal of the vertebral column?
A. External auditory meatus (EAM)
B. Foramen magnum
C. Sella turcica
D. Crista galli

_____ 3. When taking a posteroanterior (PA) axial projection (Caldwell method) of the skull, the central ray is directed:
A. 15 degrees cephalad.
B. 15 degrees caudad.
C. 30 degrees cephalad.
D. 30 degrees caudad.

_____ 4. Which radiographic baseline is used to position the PA axial projection (Caldwell method) of the cranium?
A. Either the orbitomeatal line (OML) or the infraorbitomeatal line (IOML) can be used
B. The mentomeatal line
C. The IOML
D. The OML

5. Which cranial projection best demonstrates the occipital bone?
   A. PA
   B. PA axial (Caldwell method)
   C. Anteroposterior (AP) axial (Towne method)
   D. Lateral

6. The patient is in a prone oblique position with the midsagittal plane of the head parallel to the image receptor (IR) and the interpupillary line perpendicular to the IR. The central ray is directed perpendicularly to enter 2 inches superior to the EAM. What projection of the cranium will be demonstrated on the radiograph?
   A. Lateral
   B. AP axial (Towne method)
   C. PA axial (Caldwell method)
   D. PA

7. The patient is positioned supine with the midsagittal plane and OML perpendicular to the IR. The central ray is angled 30 degrees caudad and enters the midsagittal plane at approximately 2.5 inches superior to the glabella. What projection will be imaged on the radiograph?
   A. Lateral
   B. PA axial (Caldwell method)
   C. PA
   D. AP axial (Towne method)

8. What positioning accessory can be used to assist the patient in holding the correct position for an AP axial projection of the skull?
   A. A lead mask
   B. A wedge sponge
   C. A wedge filter
   D. An Angiliner

9. Air-filled cavities located in some bones of the face and cranium are called:
   A. cranial sutures.
   B. zygomatic prominences.
   C. paranasal sinuses.
   D. paranasal foramina.

10. Which of the following bones contain paranasal sinuses?
    1. Frontal
    2. Ethmoid
    3. Temporal
    A. 1 and 2 only
    B. 1 and 3 only
    C. 2 and 3 only
    D. 1, 2, and 3

11. What is the purpose of performing sinus radiography with the patient in the upright position?
    A. To demonstrate air–fluid levels
    B. For ease of patient positioning
    C. To prevent superimposition of the cranial structures on the paranasal sinuses
    D. Sinus radiography does not have to be performed with the patient upright

12. Which paranasal sinuses are best demonstrated in the PA axial projection (Caldwell method)?
    1. Maxillary
    2. Frontal
    3. Ethmoid
    A. 1 and 2 only
    B. 1 and 3 only
    C. 2 and 3 only
    D. 1, 2, and 3

13. Which of the following projections will demonstrate the sphenoid sinus?
    A. Parietoacanthial (Waters method)
    B. Lateral
    C. AP axial (Towne method)
    D. PA axial (Caldwell method)

14. Which projection best demonstrates the maxillary sinuses?
    A. Parietoacanthial (Waters method)
    B. Submentovertex (SMV)
    C. PA axial (Caldwell method)
    D. AP axial (Towne method)

15. Which paranasal sinuses are demonstrated by the SMV projection?
    1. Sphenoid
    2. Ethmoid
    3. Maxillary
    A. 1 and 2 only
    B. 1 and 3 only
    C. 2 and 3 only
    D. 1, 2, and 3

16. Which projection will demonstrate all of the paranasal sinuses?
    A. PA axial (Caldwell method)
    B. Parietoacanthial (Waters method)
    C. Lateral
    D. SMV

17. What is the medical term for the bony sockets that house the eyes?
    A. Eye sockets
    B. Supraorbital margins
    C. Glabella
    D. Orbits

_____ 18. A lateral projection of the face using a high-resolution IR tabletop (nongrid) is used to demonstrate the:
   A. mandible.
   B. zygoma.
   C. orbits.
   D. nasal bones.

_____ 19. Which projection of the facial bones requires the central ray to exit the acanthion?
   A. AP axial (Towne method)
   B. PA axial (Caldwell method)
   C. Lateral
   D. Parietoacanthial (Waters method)

_____ 20. What is the proper central ray angle and direction for the axiolateral projection of the mandible when the midsagittal plane of the head is angled 15 degrees toward the IR?
   A. 10 degrees cephalad
   B. 10 degrees caudad
   C. 25 degrees cephalad
   D. 25 degrees caudad

Simulated Examination for the Limited Scope of Practice in Radiography—Skull/Sinuses Module

Answer Section

Multiple Choice

1. **ANS: C**	REF: Ch. 17	OBJ: exam spec E.3.A.2	TOP: skull anatomy
2. **ANS: B**	REF: Ch. 17	OBJ: exam spec E.3.A.2	TOP: skull anatomy
3. **ANS: B**	REF: Ch. 17	OBJ: exam spec E.3.A.2	TOP: skull anatomy
4. **ANS: D**	REF: Ch. 17	OBJ: exam spec E.3.A.1	TOP: skull positioning
5. **ANS: C**	REF: Ch. 17	OBJ: exam spec E.3.A.1	TOP: skull positioning
6. **ANS: A**	REF: Ch. 17	OBJ: exam spec E.3.A.1	TOP: skull positioning
7. **ANS: D**	REF: Ch. 17	OBJ: exam spec E.3.A.1	TOP: skull positioning
8. **ANS: C**	REF: Ch. 17	OBJ: exam spec E.3.A.4	TOP: skull positioning accessory
9. **ANS: C**	REF: Ch. 17	OBJ: exam spec E.3.B.2	TOP: sinus anatomy
10. **ANS: A**	REF: Ch. 17	OBJ: exam spec E.3.B.2	TOP: sinus anatomy
11. **ANS: A**	REF: Ch. 17	OBJ: exam spec E.3.B.3	TOP: sinus technique
12. **ANS: C**	REF: Ch. 17	OBJ: exam spec E.3.B.1	TOP: sinus positioning
13. **ANS: B**	REF: Ch. 17	OBJ: exam spec E.3.B.1	TOP: sinus positioning
14. **ANS: A**	REF: Ch. 17	OBJ: exam spec E.3.B.1	TOP: sinus positioning
15. **ANS: A**	REF: Ch. 17	OBJ: exam spec E.3.B.1	TOP: sinus positioning
16. **ANS: C**	REF: Ch. 17	OBJ: exam spec E.3.B.1	TOP: sinus positioning
17. **ANS: D**	REF: Ch. 17	OBJ: exam spec E.3.C.2	TOP: facial bones anatomy
18. **ANS: D**	REF: Ch. 17	OBJ: exam spec E.3.C.1	TOP: facial bones positioning
19. **ANS: D**	REF: Ch. 17	OBJ: exam spec E.3.C.1	TOP: facial bones positioning
20. **ANS: A**	REF: Ch. 17	OBJ: exam spec E.3.C.1	TOP: facial bones positioning

Complete this examination in pencil if you plan to take it more than once. If you are not sure of the answer to a question, skip it and return to it after completing the entire examination.

Multiple Choice

Identify the choice that best completes the statement or answers the question.

_____ 1. How many vertebrae are located in the cervical region of the spine?
A. 5
B. 12
C. 7
D. 9

_____ 2. What is the odontoid process and where is it located?
A. A sharp process on the inferior surface of C1
B. A toothlike projection on the superior surface of C2
C. A rounded prominence on the posterior aspect of C7
D. A palpable landmark on the mandible

_____ 3. When taking an anteroposterior (AP) axial projection of the cervical spine, the central ray is directed:
A. 15 degrees caudad.
B. 15 degrees cephalad.
C. 25 degrees caudad.
D. 25 degrees cephalad.

_____ 4. What is the rationale for using a 72-inch source–image receptor distance (SID) for the lateral projection of the cervical spine?
A. This SID enables the limited operator to use a technique with lower kilovoltage (kVp).
B. This SID reduces the patient dose.
C. This SID helps to overcome the magnification caused by the increased object–image receptor distance (OID) of the position.
D. This SID provides more room for the limited operator to assist the patient in getting into the proper position.

_____ 5. What anatomic structures of the cervical spine are best demonstrated by the lateral projection?
A. Intervertebral disks
B. Intervertebral foramina
C. Zygapophyseal joints
D. Pedicles

_____ 6. What is the proper central ray angle and direction for the AP oblique projections of the cervical spine?
A. 15 degrees cephalad
B. 15 degrees caudad
C. 45 degrees cephalad
D. 45 degrees caudad

_____ 7. What is the proper patient position for an AP oblique projection of the cervical spine?
A. 45-degree posterior oblique position
B. 45-degree anterior oblique position
C. Coronal plane positioned parallel to the image receptor (IR)
D. Supine with the base of the skull aligned with the edges of the front teeth

_____ 8. What anatomic structures are best demonstrated by the posteroanterior (PA) oblique projections of the cervical spine?
A. Zygapophyseal joints closer to the IR
B. Zygapophyseal joints farther from the IR
C. Intervertebral foramina closer to the IR
D. Intervertebral foramina farther from the IR

_____ 9. How many vertebrae make up the thoracic spine?
A. 5
B. 7
C. 12
D. 22

_____ 10. Which vertebrae have special facets for articulation with the ribs?
A. Cervical
B. Thoracic
C. Lumbar
D. Sacral

_____ 11. Breathing technique is used to advantage when taking a lateral projection of the:
A. cervical spine.
B. thoracic spine.
C. lumbar spine.
D. sacrum.

_____ 12. The patient is positioned with the coronal plane of the body perpendicular to the IR, the midsagittal plane parallel to the IR, and the arm closest to the IR raised over the head. The central ray is perpendicular and centered to the level of the C7 to T1 interspace. What projection and anatomy will be demonstrated in this image?
A. A lateral projection of the cervicothoracic region
B. An AP projection of the lower cervical spine
C. A lateral projection of the lower cervical spine
D. An AP projection of the cervicothoracic region

6. When taking an anteroposterior (AP) axial projection of the foot, the central ray is directed:
   A. 10 degrees toward the toes.
   B. 10 degrees toward the heel.
   C. 25 degrees toward the heel.
   D. perpendicular to the image receptor (IR).

7. Where does the central ray enter the patient for the AP axial projection of the foot?
   A. At the third MTP joint
   B. At the first MTP joint
   C. At the base of the third metatarsal
   D. At the head of the third metatarsal

8. Which surface of the foot should be in contact with the IR for the recumbent lateral projection of the foot?
   A. Lateral
   B. Medial
   C. Dorsal
   D. Plantar

9. Which of the following is true regarding the lateral projection of the foot?
   A. The ankle does not have a specific position when a lateral projection of the foot is performed.
   B. The ankle should be dorsiflexed so that the long axis of the foot forms a 45-degree angle with the tibia.
   C. The ankle should be extended so that the plantar surface of the foot forms a 45-degree angle with the IR.
   D. The ankle should be dorsiflexed so that the long axis of the foot is perpendicular to the tibia.

10. How much is the plantar surface of the foot elevated from the IR for the AP oblique projection of the foot?
    A. 45 degrees
    B. 30 degrees
    C. 10 degrees
    D. 25 degrees

11. Which foot projection and position will demonstrate the metatarsals (third through fifth) without superimposition?
    A. AP axial projection with the plantar surface of the foot in contact with the IR
    B. AP oblique projection in 30-degree lateral rotation
    C. AP oblique projection in 30-degree medial rotation
    D. Lateral projection with the MTP joints perpendicular to the IR

12. Which foot projection and position will demonstrate the medial and intermediate cuneiforms without superimposition?
    A. AP axial projection with the plantar surface of the foot in contact with the IR
    B. AP oblique projection in 30-degree lateral rotation
    C. AP oblique projection in 30-degree medial rotation
    D. Lateral projection with the MTP joints perpendicular to the IR

13. Which foot projection and position will demonstrate the cuboid, navicular, and lateral cuneiforms without superimposition?
    A. AP axial projection with the plantar surface of the foot in contact with the IR
    B. AP oblique projection in 30-degree lateral rotation
    C. AP oblique projection in 30-degree medial rotation
    D. Lateral projection with the MTP joints perpendicular to the IR

14. Which foot projection and position will demonstrate the entire foot in near anatomic position?
    A. AP axial projection with the plantar surface of the foot in contact with the IR
    B. AP oblique projection in 30-degree lateral rotation
    C. AP oblique projection in 30-degree medial rotation
    D. Lateral projection with the MTP joints perpendicular to the IR

15. What is the name given to the distal end of the fibula?
    A. Talus
    B. Medial malleolus
    C. Lateral malleolus
    D. Astragalus

16. Which of the following are the bones that articulate to form the ankle mortise?
    A. Talus, tibia, and fibula
    B. Tibia, fibula, and calcaneus
    C. Talus and tibia
    D. Calcaneus and tibia

17. When the leg is extended, the ankle is dorsiflexed to form an angle of 90 degrees between the foot and leg, the leg is rotated medially approximately 15 degrees, and the central ray is perpendicular to the IR through the midpoint between the malleoli, the resulting image will demonstrate:
   A. an axial projection of the calcaneus.
   B. an AP projection of the tarsals and metatarsals.
   C. the ankle mortise, especially the talofibular articulation.
   D. the cuboid and the third cuneiform.

18. Where should the central ray enter the patient for the AP projection of the ankle joint?
   A. Perpendicular to a point midway between the malleoli
   B. Perpendicular to the base of the third metatarsal
   C. Angled 10 degrees cephalad to a point midway between the malleoli
   D. Angled 10 degrees cephalad to the base of the third metatarsal

19. Which surface of the ankle is placed in contact with the IR for the upright lateral projection of the ankle?
   A. Medial surface
   B. Lateral surface
   C. Anterior surface
   D. Posterior surface

20. What is the proper central ray angle and direction for the axial projection of the calcaneus when the ankle is dorsiflexed so that the plantar surface of the foot is perpendicular to the IR?
   A. 10 degrees cephalad
   B. 40 degrees cephalad
   C. 10 degrees caudad
   D. 40 degrees caudad

Simulated Examination for the Limited Scope of Practice in Radiography—Podiatry Module

Answer Section

Multiple Choice

1. **ANS: C**	REF: Ch. 14	OBJ: exam spec E.5.A.2	TOP: foot anatomy
2. **ANS: B**	REF: Ch. 14	OBJ: exam spec E.5.A.2	TOP: foot anatomy
3. **ANS: D**	REF: Ch. 14	OBJ: exam spec E.5.A.2	TOP: foot anatomy
4. **ANS: D**	REF: Ch. 14	OBJ: exam spec E.5.A.2	TOP: foot anatomy
5. **ANS: A**	REF: Ch. 14	OBJ: exam spec E.5.A.2	TOP: foot anatomy
6. **ANS: B**	REF: Ch. 14	OBJ: exam spec E.5.A.1	TOP: foot positioning
7. **ANS: C**	REF: Ch. 14	OBJ: exam spec E.5.A.1	TOP: foot positioning
8. **ANS: A**	REF: Ch. 14	OBJ: exam spec E.5.A.1	TOP: foot positioning
9. **ANS: D**	REF: Ch. 14	OBJ: exam spec E.5.A.1	TOP: foot positioning
10. **ANS: B**	REF: Ch. 14	OBJ: exam spec E.5.A.1	TOP: foot positioning
11. **ANS: C**	REF: Ch. 14	OBJ: exam spec E.5.A.1	TOP: foot positioning
12. **ANS: B**	REF: Ch. 14	OBJ: exam spec E.5.A.1	TOP: foot positioning
13. **ANS: C**	REF: Ch. 14	OBJ: exam spec E.5.A.1	TOP: foot positioning
14. **ANS: A**	REF: Ch. 14	OBJ: exam spec E.5.A.1	TOP: foot positioning
15. **ANS: C**	REF: Ch. 14	OBJ: exam spec E.5.B.2	TOP: ankle anatomy
16. **ANS: A**	REF: Ch. 14	OBJ: exam spec E.5.B.2	TOP: ankle anatomy
17. **ANS: C**	REF: Ch. 14	OBJ: exam spec E.5.B.1	TOP: ankle positioning
18. **ANS: A**	REF: Ch. 14	OBJ: exam spec E.5.B.1	TOP: ankle positioning
19. **ANS: A**	REF: Ch. 14	OBJ: exam spec E.5.B.1	TOP: ankle positioning
20. **ANS: B**	REF: Ch. 14	OBJ: exam spec E.5.C.1	TOP: calcaneus positioning

Introduction

This guide is provided to help you prepare to successfully complete the licensure examination for the limited scope of practice area in which you are or will be working. We have included helpful suggestions for optimizing your study time and a simulated practice examination to help identify your areas of strength and weakness. All suggestions and discussions are based on the American Registry of Radiologic Technologists (ARRT) Content Specifications for the Bone Densitometry Equipment Operators Examination. We have done this for two reasons: first, this is a comprehensive examination covering all relevant areas of practice, and, second, it is likely that the licensure agency in your state uses this examination. If your state does not use this examination, you will still be well prepared if you use the ARRT Content Specifications as your study guide. For your convenience, we have included the most recent ARRT Content Specifications in this guide.

If you are using *Radiography Essentials for Limited Practice* and this accompanying workbook, it is likely that you are participating in an educational program designed to prepare you to both work in the practice area and to successfully pass the appropriate state licensure examination. This guide should assist you in both of these areas. Completing the simulated examination will help identify knowledge you have already acquired and knowledge that you have yet to master. Because the simulated examination was constructed to assess content identified in the ARRT Content Specifications, it is appropriate to provide an overview of this document before moving on to the examination.

The ARRT Content Specifications for the Bone Densitometry Equipment Operators Examination covers six content areas. These include basic concepts, equipment operation radiation safety, and dual-energy x-ray absorptiometry (DXA) scanning of the forearm, lumbar spine, and proximal femur.

The most valuable component of the Content Specifications is the outline of each content area covered on the examination. The numbers in parentheses indicate how many questions on the examination assess some aspect of that knowledge area. The value to you is that this information will help you determine how much time and effort

to spend on certain topics. Without using this information as a guide, you may waste valuable time learning information that is not included in the examination. However, we are not suggesting that you deviate from the curriculum established by your state agency or by your teacher. This guide is to help you prepare for the state licensure examination, not to prepare you to work in your practice area. You will need skills that cannot be directly assessed on a written examination.

The Simulated Examination for Bone Densitometry Equipment Operators Licensure is located after the ARRT Content Specifications in this section. You should schedule enough time to complete the entire examination at one sitting. This will give you experience in completing an examination of the length of the simulated examination and will also give you some idea of how much time you will need for this examination.

The simulated examination consists of 60 questions, as prescribed in the ARRT Content Specifications, and contains the appropriate number of questions from each of the six content areas: basic concepts (10); equipment operation (15); radiation safety (9); and DXA scanning of the forearm (6), lumbar spine (10), and proximal femur (10). The questions are further focused to cover content topics specified in the outline for each content area. You will see that there are more content topics in each outline than there are questions included in the examination. This means that some content will not be assessed with a question on both the simulated examination and your actual state licensure examination. For this reason it is important for you to review all topics included in each content outline in the ARRT Content Specifications. You cannot rely only on the simulated examination to prepare you for your state licensure examination.

The answers to all simulated examination questions are located after the last question. We have included the correct answer (ANS), as well as the *Radiography Essentials for Limited Practice* textbook chapter (REF) where the information is located, the ARRT Content Specifications topic outline designator (OBJ) that the question is designed to assess, and the topic (TOP) assessed by each question. This information will allow you to easily find and review text material that you have not yet mastered.

279

Introduction

E. DXA SCANNING OF LUMBAR SPINE (10)

1. **Anatomy**
   a. Regions of Interest
   b. Bony Landmarks
   c. Radiographic Appearance
   d. Adjacent Structures

2. **Scan Acquisition**
   a. Patient Instructions
   b. Patient Positioning
   c. Evaluating Pre-Set Scan Parameters

3. **Scan Analysis and Printout**
   a. Accurate ROI Placement
   b. BMC, Area, and BMD
   c. T-score, Z-score

4. **Common Problems**
   a. Poor Bone Edge Detection
   b. Nonremovable Artifacts
   c. Variant Anatomy
   d. Fractures or Pathology

5. **Follow-Up Scans**
   a. Unit of Comparison
      1. BMD
      2. T-score
   b. Reproduce Baseline Study

F. DXA SCANNING OF PROXIMAL FEMUR (10)

1. **Anatomy**
   a. Regions of Interest
   b. Bony Landmarks
   c. Radiographic Appearance
   d. Adjacent Structures

2. **Scan Acquisition**
   a. Patient Instructions
   b. Patient Positioning
   c. Evaluating Pre-Set Scan Parameters

3. **Scan Analysis and Printout**
   a. Accurate ROI Placement
   b. BMC, Area, and BMD
   c. T-score, Z-score

4. **Common Problems**
   a. Poor Bone Edge Detection
   b. Nonremovable Artifacts
   c. Variant Anatomy
   d. Fractures or Pathology

5. **Follow-Up Scans**
   a. Unit of Comparison
      1. BMD
      2. T-score
   b. Reproduce Baseline Study

Simulated Examination for Bone Densitometry Equipment Operator Licensure

SIMULATED EXAMINATION FOR BONE DENSITOMETRY EQUIPMENT OPERATOR LICENSURE

Complete this examination in pencil if you plan to take it more than once. If you are not sure of the answer to a question, skip it and return to it after completing the entire examination.

Multiple Choice
Identify the choice that best completes the statement or answers the question.

BASIC CONCEPTS (10)

_____ 1. According to the World Health Organization (WHO), what T-score level indicates osteoporosis?
A. +1 to −1
B. −1 to −2.5
C. −2.5 or less
D. −1 or greater

_____ 2. Primary type I osteoporosis is classified as:
A. premenopausal.
B. postmenopausal.
C. senile.
D. rheumatoid.

_____ 3. Which of the following is an uncontrollable risk factor for osteoporosis?
A. Gender
B. Estrogen deficiency
C. Low calcium intake
D. Smoking

_____ 4. What are the two basic types of bone?
A. Cortical and trabecular
B. Cortical and compact
C. Trabecular and cancellous
D. Trabecular and os calcis

_____ 5. Which of the following cells are responsible for building bone?
A. Osteotytes
B. Osteolytes
C. Osteoclasts
D. Osteoblasts

_____ 6. Bone health requires adequate intake and absorption of what two substances?
A. Calcium and potassium
B. Calcium and vitamin D
C. Potassium and vitamin D
D. Vitamin D and vitamin E

_____ 7. Two common conditions known to cause secondary osteoporosis are:
A. hyperparathyroidism and rheumatoid arthritis.
B. hyperlipidemia and rheumatoid arthritis.
C. hyperlipidemia and hyperparathyroidism.
D. rheumatoid arthritis and osteoarthritis.

_____ 8. Two weight-bearing types of exercise important for building and maintaining bone mass are:
A. swimming and jogging.
B. swimming and dancing.
C. dancing and jogging.
D. dancing and bicycling.

_____ 9. Three controllable risk factors for osteoporosis include:
A. smoking, alcohol, and calcium.
B. smoking, alcohol, and age.
C. smoking, gender, and calcium.
D. smoking, gender, and alcohol.

_____ 10. Trabecular bone accounts for what percentage of the skeletal mass?
A. 10%
B. 20%
C. 30%
D. 40%

EQUIPMENT OPERATION (15)

_____ 11. Which BMD testing method is considered the "gold standard" for diagnosis and monitoring of osteoporosis?
A. QUS
B. RA
C. SXA
D. DXA

12. What does BMD stand for, as it relates to osteoporosis testing?
    A. Body mass determination
    B. Bone mineral density
    C. Bone muscle distribution
    D. Biomass density

13. Which BMD measurement score indicates the number of standard deviations (SDs) from the average BMD of young, normal, gender-matched individuals with peak bone mass?
    A. T-score
    B. W-score
    C. V-score
    D. Z-score

14. Which BMD measurement score indicates the number of SDs from the average BMD for the patient's respective age group and gender group?
    A. T-score
    B. W-score
    C. V-score
    D. Z-score

15. Which prime factor of x-ray production controls the quality or penetrating property?
    A. mA
    B. mAs
    C. S
    D. kVp

16. Which prime factor of x-ray production controls the quantity or intensity property?
    A. mA
    B. S
    C. kVp
    D. Filtration

17. DXA bone densitometry requires how many photon energy levels?
    A. One
    B. Two
    C. Three
    D. Four

18. Which quantitative performance measure is most important in following a patient's BMD over time?
    A. Stability
    B. Accuracy
    C. Geometry
    D. Precision

19. Scanner quality control to detect shift or drift is accomplished by imaging what object?
    A. Phantom
    B. Filter
    C. Grid
    D. Patient

20. On a normal functioning scanner, when should daily scanner quality control be performed?
    A. Before the first patient
    B. Between every patient
    C. Between every fifth and sixth patient
    D. After the last patient only

21. In order to adequately preserve scan files and data, which daily computer procedures are recommended?
    A. Locate and restore
    B. Locate and backup
    C. Backup and archive
    D. Backup and restore

22. In how many directions does an array or fan-beam DXA scanner system travel?
    A. One
    B. Two
    C. Three
    D. Four

23. What is the formula for determining BMD?
    A. BMD = BMC/Area
    B. BMD = BMD/BMC
    C. BMD = Area/BMD
    D. BMD = BMC/BMD

24. What is the purpose of the FRAX tool?
    A. Monitor phantom scan
    B. Monitor bone mass
    C. Evaluate 10-year machine accuracy
    D. Evaluate 10-year fracture risk

25. Vertebral fracture assessment (VFA) is performed for what purpose?
    A. Detect bone mass
    B. Detect fractures
    C. Detect osteoporosis
    D. Detect osteopenia

RADIATION SAFETY (9)

26. What does the radiation protection principle ALARA stand for?
    A. As long as reasonably allowed
    B. As long as realistically achievable
    C. As low as reasonably achievable
    D. As low as realistically allowed

27. What are the three basic methods of minimizing radiation exposure?
    A. Time, distance, and shielding
    B. Time, distance, and monitoring
    C. Time, exposure, and monitoring
    D. Time, exposure, and shielding

28. What is the unit of absorbed dose, in addition to rad?
    A. Rem
    B. Sievert
    C. Gray
    D. Roentgen

29. What is the unit of effective dose (equivalent), in addition to rem?
    A. Rad
    B. Sievert
    C. Gray
    D. Roentgen

30. Which of the following will be the highest radiation source?
    A. Posteroanterior (PA) chest radiograph
    B. Round-trip cross-country airline flight
    C. Daily natural background radiation
    D. DXA scan of the forearm

31. Which of the following will be the lowest radiation source?
    A. PA chest radiograph
    B. Round-trip cross-country airline flight
    C. Daily natural background radiation
    D. DXA scan of the forearm

32. Which of the following is a potential long-term effect of radiation exposure?
    A. Cancer
    B. Skin reddening
    C. Significant, rapid hair loss
    D. Sudden intestinal bleeding

33. For maximum radiation protection, the suggested distance between an array or fan-beam scanner source and the operator is:
    A. 3 feet.
    B. 6 feet.
    C. 9 feet.
    D. 12 feet.

34. Patients should be screened at scheduling to avoid unnecessary radiation exposure. Contraindications for a central DXA scan would include:
    A. recent chest x-ray.
    B. recent mammogram.
    C. recent barium examination.
    D. recent lumbar spine x-ray.

DXA SCANNING OF THE FOREARM (6)

35. Which forearm is recommended for scanning?
    A. Left
    B. Right
    C. Dominant
    D. Nondominant

36. The preferred region of interest (ROI) when analyzing the forearm is:
    A. ultradistal ulna.
    B. ultradistal radius.
    C. one-third (33%) region of the ulna.
    D. one-third (33%) region of the radius.

37. What is the most common problem in scanning a forearm?
    A. Artifacts
    B. Motion
    C. Poor edge detection
    D. Poor positioning

38. Name one contraindication to scanning the forearm.
    A. Obesity
    B. Hyperlipidemia
    C. History of radial fracture
    D. History of humeral fracture

39. When doing a forearm scan, the same chair should be used to ensure consistency over time. Name a necessary characteristic of the chair.
    A. No wheels
    B. No padding
    C. No back
    D. No metal

40. When positioning a forearm for scanning:
    A. forearm must be straight and centered.
    B. forearm must be straight and not centered.
    C. forearm must be obliqued and centered.
    D. forearm must be obliqued and not centered.

DXA SCANNING OF THE LUMBAR SPINE (10)

41. What are the regions of interest for a lumbar spine DXA scan?
    A. T12 through L3
    B. L1 through L4
    C. L1 through L5
    D. L2 through L5

42. What positioning aid is typically used during lumbar spine DXA scanning?
    A. Positioning leg block
    B. Positioning spine block
    C. Gonad shielding
    D. Measuring calipers

43. Which vertebra has an H or X appearance on a lumbar spine DXA scan?
    A. L2
    B. L3
    C. L4
    D. L5

Simulated Examination for Bone Densitometry Equipment Operator Licensure

44. Which of the following variant anatomic conditions can result in a falsely elevated bone mass density (BMD) measurement on lumbar spine DXA scans?
   A. Scoliosis
   B. Kyphosis
   C. Lordosis
   D. Spina bifida

45. Which lumbar vertebra commonly has the widest transverse process?
   A. L1
   B. L2
   C. L3
   D. L4

46. Which of the following can falsely elevate the BMD measurement in a lumbar spine scan?
   A. Compression fracture
   B. Motion
   C. Obesity
   D. Spina bifida

47. When analyzing a lumbar spine scan in which more than five vertebral bodies have been imaged, always analyze by:
   A. locating L1 and counting down.
   B. locating L5 and counting up.
   C. locating L2 and counting down.
   D. locating L3 and counting up.

48. When scanning the lumbar spine, what is one of the external landmarks used for placement of the central ray?
   A. 2 cm below the greater trochanter
   B. 2 cm below the iliac crest
   C. 2 cm above the greater trochanter
   D. 2 cm above the xiphoid process

49. To which scan should a serial scan of the lumbar spine be compared?
   A. Second scan
   B. Third scan
   C. Baseline scan
   D. Do not compare

50. What is the least number of vertebrae that can be used for diagnostic BMD interpretation?
   A. One
   B. Two
   C. Three
   D. Four

SCANNING OF THE PROXIMAL FEMUR (10)

51. When positioning the proximal femur, the femoral shaft is:
   A. abducted 5 to 15 degrees.
   B. abducted 15 to 25 degrees.
   C. adducted 5 to 15 degrees.
   D. adducted 15 to 25 degrees.

52. Name the two regions of interest (ROIs) for the proximal femur.
   A. Femoral neck and total hip
   B. Greater trochanter and total hip
   C. Lesser trochanter and total hip
   D. Femoral head and total hip

53. When positioning the proximal femur, the femoral neck is also:
   A. lateral with the tabletop.
   B. oblique with the tabletop.
   C. perpendicular to the tabletop.
   D. parallel with the tabletop.

54. To which scan should a serial scan of the proximal femur be compared?
   A. Baseline scan
   B. Second scan
   C. Third scan
   D. Do not compare

55. Name one contraindication to scanning the proximal femur.
   A. Hyperlipidemia
   B. Fracture of the proximal femur
   C. Fracture of the proximal humerus
   D. Appendectomy

56. Name one of the landmarks used for placement of the central ray when scanning the proximal femur.
   A. Perpendicular to the xiphoid process
   B. Perpendicular to the iliac crest
   C. 7 to 8 cm below the greater trochanter
   D. 7 to 8 cm below the lesser trochanter

57. Why is the proximal femur scan one of the most important skeletal scans in central densitometry?
   A. Best predictor of future hip fractures
   B. Best predictor of future wrist fractures
   C. Best predictor of future vertebral fractures
   D. Best predictor of future knee fractures

58. Which of the following conditions can falsely elevate the BMD in a proximal femur scan?
   A. Osteoporosis
   B. Osteoarthritis
   C. Osteopenia
   D. Osteogenesis imperfecta

_____ 59. Image analysis of a proximal femur scan must include adequate space between:
  A. greater trochanter and femoral neck.
  B. ischium and femoral neck.
  C. lesser trochanter and femoral neck.
  D. femoral head and femoral neck.

_____ 60. Image analysis of a proximal femur scan that shows a prominent lesser trochanter may indicate:
  A. osteoporosis.
  B. osteopenia.
  C. poor rotation.
  D. artifacts.

Simulated Examination for Bone Densitometry Equipment Operator Licensure

Answer Section

Multiple Choice

1. **ANS: C**	REF. Ch. 26	OBJ: exam spec A.A.1	TOP: osteoporosis
2. **ANS: B**	REF. Ch. 26	OBJ: exam spec A.1.b	TOP: osteoporosis
3. **ANS: A**	REF. Ch. 26	OBJ: exam spec A.3.2	TOP: bone health
4. **ANS: A**	REF. Ch. 26	OBJ: exam spec A.2.b	TOP: bone physiology
5. **ANS: D**	REF. Ch. 26	OBJ: exam spec A.2.C.2	TOP: bone physiology
6. **ANS: B**	REF. Ch. 26	OBJ: exam spec A.3.a	TOP: bone health
7. **ANS: A**	REF. Ch. 26	OBJ: exam spec A.1.b	TOP: osteoporosis
8. **ANS: C**	REF. Ch. 26	OBJ: exam spec A.3.b	TOP: bone health
9. **ANS: A**	REF. Ch. 26	OBJ: exam spec A.3.C.1	TOP: bone health
10. **ANS: B**	REF. Ch. 26	OBJ: exam spec A.2.B.2	TOP: bone physiology
11. **ANS: D**	REF. Ch. 26	OBJ: exam spec B.5	TOP: measuring BMD
12. **ANS: B**	REF. Ch. 26	OBJ: exam spec B.5.B.1	TOP: measuring BMD
13. **ANS: A**	REF. Ch. 26	OBJ: exam spec B.5.B.3	TOP: measuring BMD
14. **ANS: D**	REF. Ch. 26	OBJ: exam spec B.5.B.2	TOP: measuring BMD
15. **ANS: D**	REF. Ch. 26	OBJ: exam spec B.2.A.1	TOP: measuring BMD
16. **ANS: A**	REF. Ch. 26	OBJ: exam spec B.2.A.2	TOP: fundamentals of x-ray production
17. **ANS: B**	REF. Ch. 26	OBJ: exam spec B.2.c	TOP: fundamentals of x-ray production
18. **ANS: D**	REF. Ch. 26	OBJ: exam spec B.6.a	TOP: determining quality in BMD
19. **ANS: A**	REF. Ch. 26	OBJ: exam spec B.4.D.1	TOP: quality control
20. **ANS: A**	REF. Ch. 26	OBJ: exam spec B.4.d	TOP: quality control
21. **ANS: C**	REF. Ch. 26	OBJ: exam spec B.1.b	TOP: computer console
22. **ANS: A**	REF. Ch. 26	OBJ: exam spec B.3.b	TOP: types of DXA systems
23. **ANS: A**	REF. Ch. 26	OBJ: exam spec B.5.B.1	TOP: measuring BMD
24. **ANS: D**	REF. Ch. 26	OBJ: exam spec B.5.c	TOP: measuring BMD
25. **ANS: B**	REF. Ch. 26	OBJ: exam spec B.5.d	TOP: measuring BMD
26. **ANS: C**	REF. Ch. 26	OBJ: exam spec C.1.a	TOP: fundamental principles
27. **ANS: A**	REF. Ch. 26	OBJ: exam spec C.1.b	TOP: fundamental principles
28. **ANS: C**	REF. Ch. 26	OBJ: exam spec C.3.a	TOP: units of measurement
29. **ANS: B**	REF. Ch. 26	OBJ: exam spec C.3.b	TOP: units of measurement
30. **ANS: B**	REF. Ch. 26	OBJ: exam spec C.4.1.d	TOP: radiation protection in BD
31. **ANS: D**	REF. Ch. 26	OBJ: exam spec C.4.1.a	TOP: radiation protection in BD
32. **ANS: A**	REF. Ch. 26	OBJ: exam spec C.2.a	TOP: biologic effects of radiation
33. **ANS: C**	REF. Ch. 26	OBJ: exam spec C.4.B.1	TOP: radiation protection in BD
34. **ANS: C**	REF. Ch. 26	OBJ: exam spec C.4.C.2	TOP: radiation protection in BD
35. **ANS: D**	REF. Ch. 26	OBJ: exam spec D.1	TOP: anatomy
36. **ANS: D**	REF. Ch. 26	OBJ: exam spec D.3.a	TOP: scan analysis
37. **ANS: B**	REF. Ch. 26	OBJ: exam spec D.2.b	TOP: scan acquisition
38. **ANS: C**	REF. Ch. 26	OBJ: exam spec D.4.d	TOP: common problems
39. **ANS: A**	REF. Ch. 26	OBJ: exam spec D.2.1	TOP: scan acquisition
40. **ANS: A**	REF. Ch. 26	OBJ: exam spec D.2.b	TOP: scan positioning
41. **ANS: B**	REF. Ch. 26	OBJ: exam spec E.1.a	TOP: anatomy

42. **ANS: B**	REF. Ch. 26	OBJ: exam spec E.2.b	TOP: scan acquisition
43. **ANS: C**	REF. Ch. 26	OBJ: exam spec E.1.c	TOP: anatomy
44. **ANS: A**	REF. Ch. 26	OBJ: exam spec E.4.d	TOP: common problems
45. **ANS: C**	REF. Ch. 26	OBJ: exam spec E.1.c	TOP: anatomy
46. **ANS: A**	REF. Ch. 26	OBJ: exam spec E.4.d	TOP: common problems
47. **ANS: B**	REF. Ch. 26	OBJ: exam spec E.3.a	TOP: scan analysis and printout
48. **ANS: B**	REF. Ch. 26	OBJ: exam spec E.1.b	TOP: anatomy
49. **ANS: C**	REF. Ch. 26	OBJ: exam spec E.5.b	TOP: follow-up scan
50. **ANS: B**	REF. Ch. 26	OBJ: exam spec E.5.a	TOP: follow-up scan
51. **ANS: D**	REF. Ch. 26	OBJ: exam spec F.2.b	TOP: scan acquisition
52. **ANS: A**	REF. Ch. 26	OBJ: exam spec F.1.a	TOP: anatomy
53. **ANS: D**	REF. Ch. 26	OBJ: exam spec F.2.b	TOP: scan acquisition
54. **ANS: A**	REF. Ch. 26	OBJ: exam spec F.5.b	TOP: follow-up scan
55. **ANS: B**	REF. Ch. 26	OBJ: exam spec F.4.d	TOP: common problems
56. **ANS: C**	REF. Ch. 26	OBJ: exam spec F.1.b	TOP: anatomy
57. **ANS: A**	REF. Ch. 26	OBJ: exam spec F.4.d	TOP: common problems
58. **ANS: B**	REF. Ch. 26	OBJ: exam spec F.3.b	TOP: scan acquisition and printout
59. **ANS: B**	REF. Ch. 26	OBJ: exam spec F.3.a	TOP: scan acquisition and printout
60. **ANS: C**	REF. Ch. 26	OBJ: exam spec F. 2.b	TOP: scan acquisition